CONTEMPORARY COMMUNITY HEALTH SERIES

Titles in the Series

CHILD CARE WORK WITH EMOTIONALLY DISTURBED CHILDREN

CHILD CARE WORK WITH

WITH

Genevieve W. Foster
Karen Dahlberg VanderVen
Eleanore R. Kroner
Nancy Trevorrow Carbonara
George M. Cohen

University of Pittsburgh Press

EMOTIONALLY DISTURBED CHILDREN

Library of Congress Catalog Card Number 74-158185
ISBN 0-8229-3231-8
Copyright © 1972, University of Pittsburgh Press
All rights reserved
Feffer and Simons, Inc., London
Manufactured in the United States of America
Second Printing, 1975

To Guinevere S. Chambers Vitarelli

Contents

Preface

So many things can be said and need to be said about the task of the child care worker that the material seems to be inexhaustible. Excellent volumes already available—such as Morris Fritz Mayer's *A Guide for Child Care Workers*[1] and Eva Burmeister's *The Professional Houseparent*[2] —deal with some of the principles which workers in this field must master. These principles are valid for all work with children who must be cared for away from their homes, and the volumes are a must for all students of child care work, but the population that the writers clearly have in mind is that large number of children whose behavior is either approximately "normal" or disturbed in a degree that still permits them to play like normal children and in most cases to attend ordinary schools. Bettleheim's and Redl and Wineman's landmark

1. *A Guide for Child Care Workers* (New York, 1958).
2. *The Professional Houseparent* (New York, 1960). Henry Maier includes a bibliography of child care literature prior to 1963 in his article "Child Care as a Method of Social Work" in *Training for Child Care Staff* (New York: Child Welfare League of America, 1963). Notable since that date have been Eva Burmeister, *Tough Times and Tender Moments in Child Care Work* (New York and London, 1967) and Betty Margaret Flint, *The Child and the Institution: A Study of Deprivation and Recovery* (Toronto, 1966). A useful guide to discussion is Alton M. Broten, *Houseparents in Children's Institutions: A Discussion Guide* (Chapel Hill, N.C., 1962). Since this volume was completed, an excellent work has appeared by Albert E. Trieschman, James K. Whittaker, and Larry K. Brendtro, *The Other Twenty-three Hours* (Chicago, 1969). Like the Fritz Redl and Bruno Bettleheim books mentioned in footnote 3, this volume is addressed to workers who have mastered certain basic principles of child care.

volumes,[3] on the other hand, present some of the more complicated considerations that arise in the care of the most difficult
kinds of disturbed children. Such books are useful primarily to
those who are already familiar with the everyday tasks and the
necessary attitudes of the child care worker—they are for the
advanced student. But most of these hard-to-care-for children
the country over are tended by workers who have had no special
training before coming on the job. In some institutions in-service
training courses have been set up. In other places—too few but
increasing in number—more extensive training courses have been
begun, sometimes leading to a certificate or to an associate of
arts degree in child care.

It has seemed to us who offer the present handbook that there
is a great need for a presentation of "basics" to the beginner in
work with these more difficult children. Although there is a body
of practice common to the better residential and day-care centers
for such children (certainly with some variations from place to
place), most of it is conveyed to the neophyte by word of mouth.
Much of it *must* indeed be conveyed by word of mouth, since
child care work can be learned only on the job and there is no
substitute for skilled supervision of the individual worker. Nevertheless, some time can be saved if the beginning worker or the
student in child care can read what experienced workers consider good child care to be. The literature of child care has come
hitherto largely from the field of social work. This literature has
been invaluable, but more contributions are also needed from
the point of view of child development. This volume attempts
such a contribution. Like any in the field, it can say only a part
of what needs to be said. It attempts to pick up the descriptive
task where Mayer and Burmeister leave off and to apply it to a
particular population. Others may pick up where we leave off.

What is set down here is an abstraction of child care practice,
not in a single setting but in a number of settings that are inter-

3. Bruno Bettelheim, *Love Is Not Enough* (Glencoe, Ill., 1950); Bruno
Bettleheim, *The Empty Fortress* (New York, 1967). Fritz Redl and David
Wineman, *The Aggressive Child* (Glencoe, Ill., 1957).

related in the fact that their child care staff members have been associated with the programs in child development and child care at the University of Pittsburgh.[4] Over a period of years, both a graduate program leading to the master of science degree and a nondegree certificate program[5] were built up and maintained, and in time these programs came to have an impact on child-caring agencies in the community. Nor was the influence all in one direction. As graduates from both levels of the program became involved with these agencies, there was a feedback from them to the academic staff, an exchange of thinking most fruitful for all concerned.

We are dealing here only with the body of practice that has grown up around the care of emotionally disturbed children, but it is important to remember that both programs have taught the care of children as children, whether normal or exceptional.[6] By a historical accident the term *child care worker* (or *counselor* or *houseparent*) has come to be used for those workers who, in residential or day-care centers, take charge of children whose situation is in any way unusual—those children who are neglected and dependent, physically handicapped, retarded, delinquent, disturbed, or simply underprivileged, while preschool children in a nursery school or kindergarten are in the charge of *teachers*. The task, however, of caring for all these kinds of children is basically one task.

Formal education begins (hopefully) when the child enters first grade. At this point one can begin to talk about the learning process in the narrower academic sense. Teachers everywhere, however, recognize that academic learning is influenced by many

4. Now the Department of Child Development and Child Care in the School of Health Related Professions. See Guinevere S. Chambers and Genevieve W. Foster, "Toward Improved Competence in Child Care Workers: A Two-Level Program," in *Children* (September–October 1966).

5. The certificate program was established under NIMH Grant No. 5 T1 MH 7919.

6. Every graduate student came first under the influence of Dr. Margaret McFarland, one of the pioneers in the field, who taught the basic course in early child development and directed the laboratory school.

factors—physical, emotional, and economic. Adults who are caring for children below the age of formal learning or for those with unusual needs, whether they are or are not able to attend regular schools, must study the process of early development and of learning in a broader sense than the academic and in far more detail than has been the custom in most schools of education. They must consider the processes of identification, of exploration and mastery, of control-building, and of play, as they occur in the development of all children. They must consider also the effects of separation from parents, of the absence in some cases of adequate relationships, of nutritional deficiencies, of social deprivation. They must study the slow building of ego-defenses, of the complicated processes of "coping," and the effect of too great anxiety on these processes; and they must learn to try, in some cases, to help children make up belatedly for some deficiencies in early learning that may prevent not only academic achievement but satisfactory relationships with other children and ultimately with adult contemporaries.

This body of knowledge is to be mastered not just by the academically advanced child care worker, the holder of the graduate degree. True, the graduate student must study this material and more—things like administration, supervision, research method, county and state legal systems, the conduct of training sessions in group dynamics. But in some form or other, the things enumerated in the previous two paragraphs are those which the regular, average worker with children, inside or outside the academic setting, must learn to understand. They add up to a course in early child development, taught from the point of view of dynamic psychology. If the reader should think that this subject matter is too highfalutin for the average worker, let him remember that child development has always been the territory of mothers and grandmothers, of maiden aunts and baby-nurses. What is required is not academic ambition or accomplishment so much as a sort of wholeness of vision which makes it possible for the student to observe with his feelings as well as with his mind. He is asked to observe behavior even more closely than he has been accustomed to do, to reinterpret certain kinds of behavior in the light of greater knowledge. He can learn to see the signs of anxiety in a child fully as readily as the graduate student can, and he will never forget the impact of abandonment or deprivation on a child once he has really seen it.

The study of normal child development should not be too hard to provide in most parts of the country today. Teachers well trained in this field are available, although not yet in great supply, and there are excellent texts.[7] Workers who are to have charge of disturbed children also need some additional study and experience. They need some familiarity with the different kinds of problems that can arise from physical causes or from anxiety and deprivation, and they need supervised practical work with both normal and disturbed children. This manual is offered as a supplement to the theoretical and practical study. Child care cannot be learned from a book, but a book can save the beginning worker time and uncertainty. The meaning of behavior comes only with intense striving toward understanding, based on introspective work as well as empathic observation and theoretical study. The passage that the student reads one evening can have added meaning when he rereads it the next evening if in the meantime he has been exposed to baffling behavior that is discussed on the printed page. If on the following day he approaches the same behavior with this fresh insight, he may be surprised at his own success.

The preparation of this handbook has of necessity involved a collaborative effort. The organization of the volume and the writing of most of the first two parts, with editorial revision of the whole, have been the responsibility of the senior author. Mrs. VanderVen has undertaken the writing of Parts III and IV and thus is responsible for a long section of the book. The association in the writing project of Mrs. Kroner, Mrs. Carbonara, and Mr. Cohen, all of whom have provided a great variety of philosophi-

7. L. Joseph Stone and Joseph Church, *Childhood and Adolescence* (New York, 1957); R. C. Smart and N. Smart, *Children: Development and Relationships* (New York: Macmillan Co., 1967).

cal approaches and fresh anecdotal material as they helped to enlarge and rewrite the content, has provided both a richer and a broader presentation than would have been possible otherwise. The table of contents shows their areas of responsibility. The bibliography at the end of the volume has been Mr. Cohen's contribution.

Parts II and III, "Basic Practice: Child Care Work in the Small Treatment Group" and "Child Care Work in the Large Institution," are not mutually exclusive. Child care workers in either the small or the large setting will find much in both parts that is applicable to their work. Ideally, even in large institutions, groups should be small enough and workers numerous enough and sufficiently trained to permit the more psychological approach outlined in Part II. Since this is now so far from the case, workers can still do much by emphasizing program and by such reliance on individual understanding as is possible with large numbers of children and few workers. But program is also important in its own right. As Mrs. VanderVen points out, many highly trained child care workers, well schooled in "understanding" the child, fail to understand the therapeutic value of a well-arranged game of Ping-Pong or a carpentry lesson. Without program children are thrown back on their symptomatic behavior.

Part IV, "Activity Programming," we believe will be useful to workers in both small and large settings.

The reader will occasionally find a precept repeated, sometimes more than once. This is not due to inadvertence; we have edited out those repetitions which we thought were unnecessary. But with subject matter of such complexity the reader cannot always be expected to carry over an idea or a principle into a different context. Several topics appear twice, once in relation to the small treatment group and a second time in relation to the institution. Limit-setting, for instance, is discussed in Part II and the rather more formal "discipline" in Part III. Although there is a consonance of spirit among the writers, the setting forces a different set of considerations in each case, and neither discussion would have served to cover the other situation.

It is fitting that a handbook of child care should be collaboratively written, for child care itself is always a collaborative effort if it is to be successful. All participants in the task of child care must be knowledgeable, responsible, and respected. This is not to deny the most crucial decisions to the most highly qualified professional, who in most centers is the child psychiatrist, but to assert the simple truth that those who are most closely and constantly with the child exert the decisive influence. The occupational identity of the child care worker is a new one. In the past, competent and often gifted child care workers have come from the ranks of social work, nursing, education and elsewhere. In these cases child care training has been superimposed, usually informally, on another professional skill. Others without previous training have by on-the-job experience and in-service training reached the level of certificated workers and have occasionally attained recognition as professionals. Surely trained child care workers, used to collaboration, will neither fail to recognize the genuine skills of these others nor think of them as rivals; all the workers together, from all possible sources, cannot begin to fill the needs of the children in any imaginable future. Conversely, child care can expect to be accepted by the other professions without undue jealousy. To those people (a dwindling number) who hold that disturbed children can be cared for *only* by holders of teaching certificates, *only* by hospital attendants supervised by graduate nurses, *only* by houseparents supervised by social workers, child care workers can only say: we have news for you. The shortest route to the adequate care of children is direct preparation for that task.

＊　　＊　　＊　　＊　　＊

The writers particularly wish to thank Dr. Lloyd Bell and Miss Eleanore Barovitch, who so generously contributed from their own anecdotal material for the presentation in Part II. Our thanks go also to Dr. Henry Brosin, who encouraged the writing at its beginning. Dr. Guinevere Chambers, who not only encouraged us but in a sense rode herd on the manuscript until it was ready, to the great sorrow of all of us did not live to see it published. To Dr. J. Tarlton Morrow, Jr., we owe special gratitude for his sympathetic reading of our text at an early stage of its development, for his encouragement, and for his suggestions. At a later stage of the writing, Dr. Margaret McFarland read the text and responded with warm understanding and some thoughtful criticism which we have gratefully made use of. Our thanks go also to Miss Virginia Besaw, who made several suggestions for the improvement of Part II, and to Miss Jeanne Simons and Dr. John Muldoon, who each permitted us to include an anecdote from their respective settings. Karen VanderVen as the principal author of Part III makes a special acknowledgement to the late Dr. Marion G. Marshall for contributing greatly to her understanding of how to create a therapeutic milieu for the disturbed child within an institutional setting.

Several people have been helpful in the preparation of the manuscript: Miss Roberta Gruber, of the master's program of the Department of Child Development and Child Care at the University of Pittsburgh, and Mrs. Regina Zitkovic Waid and Mrs. Patricia King, of the secretarial staff, who not only typed the manuscript but transferred innumerable messages and made innumerable arrangements for the convenience of the authors. To some of us indirect assistance has come from encouraging and forbearing spouses: Ned VanderVen, Sara Cohen, and Roger Foster. Our indebtedness to the many children with whom we all have worked over the years, and our affection for them, will we hope be evident as they appear incognito in our pages.

GENEVIEVE W. FOSTER

PART I

The Child Care Worker

*by Genevieve W. Foster and
Karen Dahlberg VanderVen*

CHAPTER 1

Temperament and Training in Child Care Work

Temperament[1]

The field of child care work requires people of many different kinds. We tend to think of the child care worker as a woman, but men do well in this field; and since, for reasons that we do not understand fully, boys outnumber girls in centers for emotionally disturbed children, there is a great need for male workers. There is also need for workers of different ages. Children need different things from different people, and they will turn to a younger worker for the satisfaction of certain needs and to an older one for others. The very young worker may seem to them like an older brother or sister, someone who they can expect will play quite actively with them, whereas the worker who is older than others may be appreciated for parental or grandparental qualities. There is room in child care work for the rather shy and retiring person, so long as he is able to set limits when necessary, and for the ebullient extravert who has enough sensitivity to recognize a child's feeling. Not all people who feel that they "love children," however, make good child care workers. The person who undertakes to work with emotionally disturbed, delinquent,

1. On this subject see *Training for Child Care Staff* (New York: Child Welfare League of America, 1963); Hyman Grossbard, *Cottage Parents: What They Have to Be, Know, and Do* (New York, 1960); Van G. Hromodka, "How Child Care Workers Are Trained in Europe," *Children* (November–December 1964); and Van G. Hromodka, "Toward Improved Competence in Child Care Workers: A look at What They Do," *Children* (September–October 1966); as well as the article cited in footnote 4 of the Preface describing the Pittsburgh programs in the same issue of *Children*.

or even just neglected and dependent children with the idea of giving tender loving care to some unfortunate child and receiving love and gratitude in return is likely to be disappointed. True, the children do often come to love the workers, but often also they are angry and defiant with them. There has usually been too much deprivation or other injury for the children to have normally affectionate feelings toward adults. The worker has to be able to appreciate the child in spite of some behavior that he finds difficult. His reward comes through seeing the child begin to grow and thrive, recover from some of his hurts, and perhaps leave the institution or treatment center to join the world of other children—and through knowing that the child's success has come about partly through his efforts.[2]

Not all workers are equally successful with all kinds of children. Some find that they relate better to young children or to very withdrawn, deeply disturbed children. Some on the other hand enjoy and can profitably use the interchange with more verbal, more active, perhaps older, perhaps "acting-out" youngsters. No one should be discouraged at the discovery that he is not equally proficient with all kinds of children; the need for child care workers is so great that a given worker can almost always find a position that suits his talents. Further, with experience one's proficiency becomes broader; the understanding of one age range or kind of disturbance sometimes leads gradually to the understanding of others.

The prospective worker need not be an intellectual, but he has to be intelligent. He will need to grasp certain parts of the theory of child development in order to perform his job adequately. His most important qualification is a certain quality of feeling—a warm spontaneous response to the child and an ability to discern what the child's feelings are. A reasonable degree of patience is necessary, as well as a tolerance for other people's

2. An unpublished but widely known paper, "Having Chosen to Work with Children," by Charlotte Babcock, M.D., of the faculty of the Pittsburgh Psychonanalytic Institute, "speaks to the condition" of those who have chosen this profession.

behavior and opinions, not only the children's but also those of one's fellow workers. Twenty years ago there were quite a few people in the field of child care of whom it was said, "She (it was usually she) doesn't get on very well with other adults, but she is wonderful with children." This kind of worker appears to be a vanishing breed. It has become fully apparent over the years that cooperating with one's fellow workers in the team effort is almost as important as working well with the children. If there is dissension among the workers, the children do not do well. Therefore, the person who has to compete too eagerly, who cannot enjoy the success of the whole team, but has to feel that he, and he alone, helped the child had better look for some other field of work where he can operate as an individual. This is not to say that the worker does not have the right to recognize and enjoy his own growing proficiency, only that child care is not a field for prima donnas, but for cooperators.

Training[3]

The single most important subject for study by the prospective child care worker is the development of the normal child. It must be studied not just as a sequence of growth and a series of changes that transform the helpless infant into an adult, but as a continuous and changing interplay between the child and the people around him, especially, in the early years, between the child and his mother or substitute mother. Some texts such as Stone and Church's *Childhood and Adolescence* and Erik H. Erikson's *Childhood and Society*[4] will introduce the student to child development in this dynamic fashion. While he is reading, however, he will need to confirm what he is learning by observing normal infants and children and if possible by helping to care for them, and to discuss what he has observed with a child development specialist. Observation of children is an art

3. See footnote 1 for pertinent resource material.
4. *Childhood and Adolescence* (New York, 1957) and *Childhood and Society* (New York, 1963).

and must be learned. The things that a trained observer can point out to an untrained one, while they are both looking at the same child or group of children, are really impressive. The student should also if possible have training in writing observations of normal children and should have the opportunity to discuss these observations with a teacher or supervisor.

The worker who will be involved with emotionally disturbed children must study the sequence of normal development carefully. But he must also know what the effects are likely to be when the child has some physical handicap or when he has been deprived of loving individual care from the beginning of his life, and what they are likely to be if separation and deprivation have occurred at various later periods of his development. The worker also needs to know something of the effects of adverse social circumstances, such as poverty so extreme that there is a real lack of stimulation. Even the "normal" children in shelters and orphanages have at the very least suffered separation from their families and friends and in many cases have also suffered neglect and rejection, even abuse. Emotionally disturbed children in large institutions, and even some of those in small treatment centers, have also in some cases suffered neglect and rejection, although in other cases they have been tenderly cared for all their lives and everything has been done for them that their parents were able to do. Nevertheless, something has gone radically wrong in the way that they feel about themselves, in their fear of things and situations that most children have learned to handle easily, and in their ability to learn. In some cases there is known to be something organically wrong with the child, but in many cases no organic damage has been demonstrated. In all these children, for whatever reason, certain kinds of interchange between the child and the mother that ordinarily take place very early have not taken place. The child care worker will find himself helping the child to go through some of these developments belatedly, when they are no longer appropriate to his age.

The interchange between a small child and his mother occurs so spontaneously and in most cases with so little apparent psycho-

logical effort, that we easily forget how complex it is. Along with
the constant physical care and protection—the feeding, the bathing, the changing, the minute-by-minute watching—a continual
teaching process is going on. The mother is introducing the child
to the world, in the most simple and material sense. She gives
him things that he can handle and mouth. She takes away things
that would hurt him or that he might damage. She encourages
him to try to do things with his hands. She is alert to his cries and
to his facial expression; if he is frightened by something she
responds immediately, and if the danger is real she removes him
or it. If it is unreal she reassures him, in words that he may perhaps not understand but whose feeling he somehow catches:
"That's only the doggie barking," "That's Daddy singing while
he shaves." Through this continual process, the small child gradually gets the idea that the world is a reasonably safe place, that
it is all right to go ahead and explore it and experiment with it,
that if something untoward happens, mother will be right there.

   While all this is going on, the mother is also conveying to the
child the feelings that he should have about himself. He only
discovers who he is—discovers that he is anybody at all in the
first place—through the feelings about him which she expresses.
In most cases, the feeling about himself that the child receives
through the mother is that he is pretty nice most of the time and
that most of what he does is pretty nice too. When he begins to
do things that she doesn't think are so nice, she lets him know,
and because of her feelings he tries to modify his behavior. With
disturbed children this process too has gone wrong. Extremely
disturbed children seem to have very little self-concept of any
sort; some of them do not use the pronoun "I" at all. Others
appear to feel that they are bad or worthless; they may not say
so in so many words, but they show it constantly in all sorts of
ways, such as trying to hurt themselves or destroying anything
that they themselves have made, especially if someone else has
admired it. An important part of the worker's task is to help the
children feel better about themselves. Telling them directly that
they are good and that the worker likes them does little good,

but it can be demonstrated day after day in the way the worker cares for them and as he helps them toward behavior and achievement that will raise their opinion of themselves. The beginning worker should learn to think of the disturbed child as one who has got stuck at some point in his psychological development, rather than as one who is simply bizarre, and to realize that most of what a disturbed child does would have been appropriate at some time in his earlier development.

Besides giving disturbed children the care that all children need, the task of the worker is thus to help them make up for lost time in mastering some of these early learning experiences that they have missed. In order to learn to perform this task, he needs to practice his art at first under the supervision of an experienced worker. There is a great difference between the disturbed child on the printed page and the child in the ward of a psychiatric hospital or day treatment center. There should be ample opportunity to discuss the student worker's interaction with the children—what they did, what he did, how the children apparently felt, how he felt, and in particular how anxious he felt. Child care is one of the arts that can be learned only in the doing. During his training period and when he begins work, the child care worker will if he is fortunate have the supervision of a child psychiatrist, with the opportunity to discuss the behavior of individual children and its meaning; or at the very least occasional psychiatric consultations should be available. This service will be available if the worker is employed in an intensive treatment center, but it is unfortunate that in many large institutions psychiatric time is scarce and most of the time the child care attendants must do the best they can without it.

In addition to his knowledge of child development and some knowledge of its deviations, the prospective worker also needs to understand a little, in a practical way, of how groups operate —how the children interact within their own group, how leadership is achieved, how some children become scapegoats, how members of a group can sometimes help one another, how the group climate can be beneficial or detrimental, and, in addition, how the interaction of the worker group affects the children. In this last respect he has to have some awareness of the way in which his own feelings affect his behavior and in which he in turn affects the children. It is helpful if a student worker can gain some of this insight during group discussions conducted by a skilled group leader. He does, however, pick up a good deal of it from the atmosphere if he is so fortunate as to work in a setting where the relationships are good and the morale high—where there is a habit of fairness and consideration, frankness in recognizing one's own occasional mistakes and acceptance of others' errors, and an absence of jealousy and backbiting.

Because he is constantly with the children, the child care worker sees and deals with much significant behavior that the "professionals" in their more peripheral roles do not. He is thus in an ideal position to make the most complete observations of the children's responses in various situations. In addition to the help that the workers give the children in their development, what they are able to pass on to others involved with the children is very important in helping the team formulate a full and accurate picture of each child's functioning. In order for the worker to be able to perform this additional aspect of his job, he should try to learn how to be a good observer and recorder of children's behavior, to be able to see and communicate the "how" and the "what" and perhaps the "why" of what the children do. Too often a day of significant behavior and meaningful child care is lost because the happenings are summed up by an "active today"; "usual self"; "spent morning in playroom," all of which contributes little insight into what the child did and how his reactions were handled. Of course, as the worker becomes more experienced in his work and broadens his basic knowledge of child development, he will become more effective in "seeing" the children and conveying his observations to others. Also, there are available works relevant to observing, such as Nancy Carbonara's *Techniques for Observing Normal Child Behavior.*[5]

5. *Techniques for Observing Normal Child Behavior* (Pittsburgh, 1961).

Finally, Dr. Robert Switzer of the Menninger Clinic, in a speech to a graduating class of child care workers, cited the importance of child care workers' having "handles"—special knowledge, interests, or skills which can be used with the children and offer an extra dimension to their lives. Children who may have had little interest in constructive activity often first develop it in response to the commitment they perceive in someone who works closely with them. A worker with a special area of interest takes on additional identity as a real person in the eyes of the children.

If the worker does not have such extras, many child care supervisors feel that at the very least it is desirable for the on-the-spot worker to be proficient in some ordinary program skill, or to develop one if he does not already bring it to the job. There is a great range of possibilities—arts and crafts, homemaking skills, games, music, sports, science, hobbies involving collection or construction. The motherly woman who can teach the adolescent girls on her unit to cook and to knit, the active young man with a fund of sports and game skills from his own childhood, the artistic young lady whose work with the children in their spare time keeps the walls covered with colorful paintings, these are workers with "handles" who enrich the lives of the children in their care. Knowledge of activities is helpful in practical management of the children as well as in broadening their range of experience and developing new skills and a sense of achievement in them. For example, boys in one treatment center still recall with excitement and pleasure evenings spent stargazing with telescopes set up by an evening worker with an interest in astronomy. These evenings might otherwise have been spent desultorily watching television or becoming increasingly hyperactive and aggressive because of boredom, thus requiring that the staff scold and restrain.

These are no small demands in the way of worker training, but they are neither unreasonable nor unattainable. Anything less in the way of training means a less benign, not to say less therapeutic, setting for disturbed children. Quite a few treatment centers have thus trained their workers, and hopefully more will do so in the future.

Responsibilities and Rights

Child care work is one of many possible jobs that are open to people who do not have college degrees. It differs from many such jobs, however, in the fact that it requires a *professional attitude* on the part of the worker. No one should go into child care work who is not capable of such an attitude. This means, first, that the worker's chief allegiance is to the children in his charge. He will do his best for them whether or not any other adult sees what he is doing. Though he has a healthy regard for his own rights, in time of emergency he will sacrifice his own convenience for the children's welfare. He, not his supervisor, is the keeper of his own conscience. He is not constantly looking for ways of getting a little extra time off, nor does he appropriate to his own use supplies that are meant for the children. He is rightly proud of his position and of his accomplishments. He is able to report honestly what has occurred between him and the children, even if it means exposing his own mistakes, and can bring his feelings (even his negative feelings) into the open when it is in the interest of the work that he should do so. While he has a strong conscience, he cannot afford to be overconventional; for he will have to learn to accept many things, both language and behavior, in the children that are unacceptable by any ordinary standards. He accepts them only provisionally, expecting that the children will change and grow, but for the time being, and perhaps for a long time to come, he has to accept them gladly.

He enters into a job situation knowing that he is going to work hard, but knowing also that his difficult task will have its own special rewards as he sees the changes in the children. He expects his hours of work and his rate of pay to be reasonable in the light of community standards for work of comparable responsibility and in consideration of any special training he has had. He can expect a reasonable amount of sick leave and paid vacation.

From his superiors in the agency or institution the worker can expect leadership and support. There must be communication on both sides. Leadership means that the philosophy of the treatment center should be made as clear as possible and constantly discussed. Whereas in some matters a clear directive must be given to the workers, for example, in the matter of a child's home visits or whether a given youngster is to be allowed outside the grounds by himself, in the subtler matters of treatment philosophy the workers must not only understand the attitude of their leaders but must agree with it; they must in fact help to shape it. There must be much give-and-take discussion with the clinical director and/or the program director (preferably with both) in order that there may be complete understanding on all sides.

Even beyond understanding, there has to be trust. As a rule the workers can implement the treatment philosophy only when they have faith in it. They may try conscientiously to carry out an order that they do not really believe in, but their lack of conviction is likely to be conveyed to the children and thus to thwart their best efforts. If the director wants them, for instance, to tolerate four-letter words and abusive language from a given child at a given time, they may grit their teeth and go along with the order, feeling all the time that what the youngster needs is a good spanking. In spite of their efforts their feeling is likely to get through to the child; he realizes that he is making them angry, and he may continue to call them more and worse names in the hope of finally getting an honest reaction from them. On the other hand, the "bad" language may for instance be serving as an outlet for a great deal of bottled-up anger that a particular child is only now able to express. If the director and the workers have thoroughly discussed the meaning of "bad" language to this child at this particular time, they can learn to convey the feeling to the child that they can accept what he is doing for the time being because he needs it, but that in time they expect him to get over it, because people do not like to be spoken to in that way. If they can say something like this to the child, he will feel relieved by their understanding of his situation and will of his own accord try to taper off his unacceptable language when the pressure of his feelings has eased.

If he is to do his best for the children, the worker will not be expected to care for too many children at once. For severely disturbed children in an intensive treatment program the usual ratio is one worker to three children at all times except when the children are sleeping, and always at least two workers to a group. When the children are less disturbed or when the worker is highly skilled at using the group process, the child-worker ratio can be higher. And there are always times of emergency, when there is much illness among the staff, when one worker will have to do his best for more children than he would prefer to care for at one time. (Children will often rise to the occasion and help the worker if they realize that the emergency is genuine.) In large institutions the ratio of staff to children is usually far less than this, and the worker in such a setting must be willing to undertake far less in the way of help to individual children. He must try by such means as program planning and group management to make up in some measure for the lack of close relationships with individual children.

In either setting the worker expects that means will be provided him to do the task that he has to do, that for instance he will have the play materials for a suitable activity program. There must be channels through which he can make his needs known, both for getting needed activity materials and for replacement and repairs.

He has to feel that a supervisory person is available to him when he needs to discuss a difficult problem that he has with a child and that there is an atmosphere in which he can discuss frankly not only his successes but his frustrations and his failures. He needs to know that help will be forthcoming and that the prevailing climate is one of understanding and of helpful criticism. To achieve an atmosphere of trust, there has to be continual communication. This means that the people in leadership positions must plan enough meetings and conferences so that everyone concerned with the children can be up to date on the latest developments in the child group and can be reasonably assured as to ways of meeting them. This subject will be further discussed in the last section of chapter 6.

Goals

Some children who are too disturbed to go to regular schools can be enabled by good child care, by individual psychotherapy when this is appropriate and available, and by skilled counseling of their parents to live at home and to go to regular schools. Four or five or even six years or longer may be required to attain this result, and then much help is often needed while the children are making their adjustment to public and private schools. Nevertheless, it can be done and would be done oftener if there were more treatment centers. Other children are too disturbed ever to mature this far. Some of these can, nevertheless, be "habilitated" enough to remain in the community, to live at home, and perhaps as they get older to hold jobs in special settings such as sheltered workshops, thus partially maintaining themselves economically. The establishment of special residential homes on the "halfway house" model, in which young people could live under supervision and go out to jobs, would enable some of them to remain in the community even if their parents could no longer care for them. Some children, of course, will not respond to any educational measures sufficiently to be kept at home as they get older. Even within institutions, however, good child care work can make such children's lives happier, more active, and more self-respecting.

CHAPTER 2

The Small Treatment Center and the Large Institution

Emotionally disturbed children include those who are so very impulsive that they cannot be placed in a group of ordinary children, those whose talk and behavior are so bizarre that they are not tolerated in ordinary groups, or those who are so withdrawn that they scarcely communicate with anybody. Such children may be those who cannot sit down in a schoolroom or play with other children without constantly disrupting what is going on, or who repeatedly run away from home, steal, set fires, or do violent things that are dangerous to others or themselves. Or they may be those who cannot go to school or play with other children because they seem to be living in an entirely different world from others; they talk but much of what they say does not make sense; they cannot be taught because nobody gets through to them. Other children, who have become disturbed when very young, have sometimes never even learned to talk, or they simply repeat back what is said to them, or say some phrase, like a television commercial, over and over. They are frequently not toilet trained; they may refuse to eat anything but certain selected foods or they may try to eat things that are harmful to them; instead of playing they may manipulate some object continually or twirl a piece of string from morning till night.

In a treatment center the diagnosis of the children's disturbance is made by a child psychiatrist with the help of a psychologist. It is their task to distinguish the children who are emotionally disturbed from those who are retarded or who have organic brain damage. Sometimes a child may be retarded or have brain damage in addition to his emotional disturbance, and sometimes the people making the diagnosis cannot be sure whether or not he has other troubles besides emotional disturbance. The diagnosis is important when psychiatric decisions are to be made, but from the child care worker's point of view a child is first of all a child, with the needs that all children have. Whatever his troubles are, he can be helped by good child care work and harmed by the lack of it.

In a treatment center, also, the child care workers have the help of a supervising or consultant child psychiatrist, who aids them in understanding each child as an individual, his special needs, and the kind of care that will help him get better. In many centers the psychiatrist meets with the child care staff at intervals, perhaps once a week. Day-to-day direction and leadership is usually given by a professional child care worker or by a psychologist, nurse, social worker, or educator who has had special training in child care. A child care worker functions not only as an individual but as a member of a team. He is in fact a member of two teams, the smaller team of child care workers and perhaps also of teachers, who are directly responsible for the children, and a larger team which includes the psychiatrist, the psychologist, and the parent counselor, who in most settings is a social worker. It is very important, if a child is to be helped, for team members to keep in close touch with one another, in order both to share information and to be sure that the efforts they are making to help the children are consistent and not in conflict. It is frequent practice for members of the child care team, and the children's teachers if there is an intramural school, to meet together at least once a day to share their experiences, concerns, and suggestions, and for the larger team to meet once a week. In addition, there may be any number of "quickie" conferences between people who need to share or settle something that cannot wait for the next formal conference. Conferences have to be managed without depriving the children of their ongoing program or of the attention they need, and this takes skillful planning. This sharing is naturally far easier in a day center where the children go home in midafternoon than in a residential center where someone must be with them constantly.

In a residential treatment center the child care staff is responsible for the children at all times except when they are in the classroom or in some other prescribed activity, such as individual psychotherapy. The worker sees them off to these activities and he catches them on the rebound. If a child has been stimulated, depressed, calmed, or made angry by his session in the schoolroom or with the psychotherapist, the child care worker receives him, recognizes his feelings, and helps him with them. The worker stands ready, if need be, to go to the schoolroom and bring back to the group room a child who on that particular day is unable to remain in class without upsetting the other children. Or if the session with the psychotherapist has been a particularly difficult one, the therapist may convey this information to one of the workers in a few words when he brings the child back, so that the workers may be alerted that special attention is needed on this occasion. In any case, school is out at two or three o'clock in the afternoon, the therapy session is over at the end of the allotted hour, but child care goes on around the clock.

The residential centers which accept the younger or more disturbed children are likely to have the child care staff working on eight-hour shifts: a morning shift from perhaps 7:00 A.M. to 3:00 P.M., an evening shift from 3:00 P.M. to 11:00 P.M., and a night shift (requiring fewer people) from 11:00 P.M. to 7:00 A.M. Other centers, which either send the children out to public schools or have an intramural school attended by all the children for a full school day, have a child care staff (usually in residence) who are responsible for the children before school in the mornings, after school in the evenings, and at nighttime, but who are free during school hours except for one or two who are on duty in rotation to take care of emergencies. Day treatment centers accept children who can live at home and attend the center from 8:30 or 9:00 A.M. till 2 or 3:00 P.M.

Each treatment center has its own staff patterns, its own routines and regulations, and its own chain of responsibility, but the basic task is always that of caring for emotionally disturbed children in such a way that they can become happier, can learn to master some of the tasks of growing up, and in fortunate cases may be able to take their place in the world of ordinary children. The worker who is caring for children who can talk and play, even though they are disturbed enough to need residential or day treatment, is naturally faced with a rather different task from that of the worker who cares for very withdrawn, nonverbal children who are not able to care for themselves or to play in the usual sense of the word. Part of the discussion in Part II applies to the more disturbed children and part to the less, but much of it applies to any child in residential or day treatment. For more extended discussions of work with children who are only moderately disturbed, the reader is referred to the manuals that are cited in the Preface.

The principles of child care are of course the same in the large setting as in the small: all the children have the same need for understanding, for communication, and for an adequate program. The very size of the large institution, however, requires special application of child care methods and of the worker's understanding of child development. The great majority of disturbed children are in the large institutions. The difficulty in institutions is that there is almost always less money to be spent per child than in the small center and each worker is therefore responsible for more children. The one-to-one contact between worker and child that is so frequent in the small center simply cannot occur so often in the institution. The worker has to adapt his methods to this circumstance; he must rely even more than the worker in the small group on planning and programming, on group techniques, and on making the contacts that he does have with each individual child as significant as possible.

The principles of child care could be better implemented if there were in every large institution smaller groups and proportionately more child care workers than there are now (but the reader will realize as he goes on that not all the advantages lie with the small center; institutions have some positive features).

Even in the present institutions, however, with their relatively too-large groups and their not-very-adequate staff coverage—in many of them at least—radical improvement can be made by the application of good child care methods. To say this is not to condone the inadequate provision of funds for disturbed children. It is necessary to move forward on more than one front. While concerned citizens make every effort to secure better financing for the care of deviant children, those who are involved with the care of the children who are presently in institutions must make as much improvement as possible in the circumstances.

What may make service in an institution especially attractive and rewarding to a child care worker is the fact that administrators in many places are trying to make the change over from *custodial* care, which means that the children are *cared for* as well as possible, to *therapeutic* care, which means that so far as possible the children are *enabled to get better* (therapy means treatment). In any large institution there will be some children who have the capacity, if they also have the opportunity, ultimately to leave the institution. Others may be able to change and develop to some extent but will always need special care and protection. Some will be capable of very little change. Within these groups, however, those who have had treatment and education will be able to lead a fuller life and in some cases even contribute to the life of the institution itself. They all need warmth and understanding; they all need good programming. It is important that every child should develop as much ego-strength as he can and that no child should deteriorate because of the inability of the institution to provide a responsive and stimulating environment.

The changeover from custodial to therapeutic care is a difficult one requiring tact, patience, and creativity on the part of many people. The administrator must balance the varying concerns of the large number of people and departments in such a way as to secure their continued involvement and interest without sacrificing therapeutic goals. In addition, he must struggle with budgetary and sometimes political difficulties. It is a continual challenge to the ingenuity and hardiness of an institutional administrator to make his program effective through the judicious use of the people and equipment that are available. Institutions tend to have a life of their own, and they are extraordinarily resistant to change. In his effort the administrator needs help at the supervisory level and especially at the level of actual work with the children. In bringing about change it is often necessary to fight the system, but in a climate of change, workers who make known to their supervisors their rational needs for improving their efforts with the children often find more support than they expect.

The physical setting of an institution may discourage the worker at first but, hopefully, will challenge him to invest his resources to improve it. The bare, long, dark corridors of some children's units, perhaps converted from adult hospital wards, often convey an atmosphere of containment, boredom, and aimlessness rather than one of activity, interest, and life. Although some newer institutions have cottages, separate buildings for each group, even some of these may have the space arranged in a way that is inappropriate to the living needs of children. Either the spaces are too large (too frightening and empty to play in except for aimless running around), or they are too small for the freedom of movement and activity that children need. Some living quarters may be too remote, so that access to appropriate activity areas is only by elevator or through several locked doors. In addition, privacy may not be possible.

In institutions also, as in many children's agencies, limited budgets may restrict the type and amount of equipment, material, and playthings available. Or through the exigencies of ordering and processing, a situation may arise such as having five gross of paintbrushes and no paint, or a playground set that can only be fastened in grass when the playground is concrete. If not that, the organization in some institutions is such that most of the play supplies are channelled to the activity departments, whereas on the living units where children still spend much time there are few play materials. Storage space for children's toys and belongings may be scarce and, if available, inappropriate for the particular children involved. All these and other problems frequently lead to a situation in which the main occupation on the living unit is watching television for the more adequate children and for the more withdrawn the aimless and perpetual manipulation of some small object.

Many institutions, unlike the small residential or day treatment centers, are like small communities, supplying for themselves many services that the smaller centers rely on the outside community to supply. For example, most large institutions run their own laundry service, maintenance department, and food service; some even generate their own electricity and make some of the items needed for everyday living. This sometimes makes for troublesome inflexibility. For instance, if the workers want to plan a picnic, they may be required to ask the dietary department for the necessary supplies a week in advance. If it rains on the appointed day, the picnic supplies will be sent up anyway, and if the following day should be fine, the picnic cannot take place because the supplies will not be forthcoming. This "community" aspect of the institution also has its positive side, which will be mentioned later.

A children's unit which is part of an adult institution often has its own special problems. The arrangements and regulations have been made for adults and often are not appropriate for children. One particularly difficult issue is the fact that all children—normal ones as well as disturbed—are naturally and necessarily in a position of dependency. The dependency of hospitalized adults is properly considered a sign of their illness, while the dependency of children is a natural component of their developmental stage. Arrangements which take this fact into account are sometimes criticized by staff outside the children's unit as "spoiling the patients." A worker in a state institution was reprimanded by the directress of nursing because she was seen crossing the grounds hand in hand with a child; this was said to be "getting too familiar with a patient." It required a vigorous argument from the unit supervisor to establish the point that any young child may have the need, and certainly has the right, to have his hand held by an adult at times.

These characteristics of some large institutions may discourage the prospective child care worker. But he can surmount his doubts if he can keep in mind the fact that he will help in bringing about a change from a custodial to a therapeutic setting, and he will find here a challenge. There is real need for his skill and understanding. His ingenuity can perhaps brighten the depressing and hospitallike setting or manipulate the space in the one that has been badly planned. He can make known the needs of the children for toys and equipment and secure the trust of his supervisors by faithfully taking care of such equipment as he is given. He can try to occupy the children constructively so that they need not spend long hours before the television or twirling objects in corners. Perhaps a surpervisor can be persuaded to mediate between the workers and the dietary staff so that the planning for picnics can be more realistic.

The positive side to the existence of community-type services within the institution is that they provide an opportunity for children to see what different adults do in the work world and perhaps even to form relationships with these adults. Creative administrators have found that properly planned associations between the children and various institutional workers have many therapeutic aspects. Also, the comprehensiveness of the institutional function may actually make many things happen more easily and faster than in smaller centers. For example, in a small setting a stopped-up sink may be a major calamity that takes hours to fix. In the large institution, a phone call to the maintenance or housekeeping department brings quick assistance.

Part III of the present volume gives a picture of some of the inevitable difficulties encountered in institutional work. It also gives the prospective child care worker a picture of how his talents can be used to help provide a truly developmental program for the children. It shows him that despite any inherent limitations there are also many possibilities open to him for doing child care work that is highly effective and that adapts itself to the weaknesses, while it utilizes the strengths, of the institutional structure.

PART II

Basic Practice: Child Care Work in the Small Treatment Group

by Genevieve W. Foster, Eleanore R. Kroner,
Nancy Trevorrow Carbonara, and George M. Cohen

CHAPTER 3

The Worker and Individual Relationships

Confidentiality

The worker will have to learn the policies of the particular agency in which he works. These are usually taught in a short period of orientation before work actually starts. One rule, however, which is common to all treatment centers is confidentiality. The names of the children must never be told to anyone outside the center, and nothing must even be mentioned about them by which they might be identified. There is a special temptation when workers are together outside the center to begin talking about their charges, but it is important to resist this temptation in all places where the conversation might be overheard, as in restaurants or elevators, or at places where other people are present.

It is important also for the workers not to talk about anything in front of the children unless they want the children included in the conversation; especially they should not discuss the children in their presence. This is true even if the children do not talk much or at all and do not seem to listen. Such children are not deaf, and they understand a great deal more than we at first suppose they do. Numerous anecdotes illustrate this point:

A child care worker once stopped another worker who was walking with a child and said, "He is having a hard time today. You'd better watch him carefully—he is 'hyper' today." As the little boy walked on with the other worker, he asked in an anxious voice, "Danny a bad boy—Danny a bad boy today?"

Communication

The worker must remember that everything he does and the way in which he does it are communications to the children. At the same time, it is important to talk *to* the children, even if they seem not to be paying attention—to tell them what the plans are for the group, who will be taking care of them if their usual worker is absent, and other things that are really of concern to them. Sometimes the worker's efforts pay off dramatically:

A boy who did not talk had to have an operation. In preparing him for surgery his worker told him what would happen and where he would go, and emphasized that he didn't have to be afraid. It was reported later that as the youngster was being made ready for the anesthetic he said, "You don't have to be afraid—these good men—they not hurt you." After repeating this he began to sing songs he had heard in the day school he attended, songs which he had never sung before. The worker's careful explanation had enabled him to comfort himself during the ordeal, although at the time it was given he had seemed not to listen.

Similar preparation is important for more usual experiences, such as a visit to the doctor or dentist or even going for a haircut. Such an event as an X ray or an electroencephalogram must be carefully explained to the child beforehand so that he will not be frightened by the strange place and people and the alarming apparatus. In a residential setting this preparation is easy to do, but even if the child is in day care, workers should know of these events and should help prepare the child for them, coordinating their efforts with those of the parents.

The possibility of communicating with extremely withdrawn, mute, and unsocialized children was a great surprise to the people who first began to work with them seriously, some twenty years ago. The beginning worker will be surprised to find himself communicating quite well with those children whose speech may be very inadequate. The child will often let the worker know by little signs what he is feeling or will respond to a request or a suggestion by his behavior, even though he cannot respond in words. The most withdrawn children often give the impression that they neither see nor hear you, that they are totally absorbed in some inner process that shuts you out completely. Nevertheless, they see and hear without seeming to do so, and if the worker is alert to their gestures, special sounds, and other signals, much communication can go on.

A mute seven-year-old, on a trip to the zoo—a trip that he had made often—suddenly refused to get off the bus at the zoo entrance. He clung to the pole at the front of the bus, and upon being detached and lifted off by the driver, he sat down on the ground and anchored one of the workers by putting an arm around each of her legs. When this worker told him he need not go to the zoo but could go back to the center, he jumped up and willingly boarded the bus again. Talking over this incident later, the workers recalled that on the previous trip to the zoo the children had seen the animals fed and that this child had been near the cage of the baby hippopotamus, who opened his mouth very wide for his dinner. They could only surmise that this experience had roused some fears in the little boy about oral aggression—that of the animals (who knows—maybe they eat little boys!) and his own (he was given to biting when he was angry). Though any such theory was guesswork, it was possible to talk to him about these fears with apparent growth on his part. Among other things, he gave up biting, and he was able again to go to the zoo.

Normal children sometimes react this way at the zoo also, but since they trust adults more, they make less of a production of it. A friend of one of the writers took a normal child to the zoo and had the same experience of seeing a hippopotamus open its mouth wide. The child said, "I'll bet he could swallow a whole boy!"

Communication of this sort with a nonverbal child is only the beginning; ultimately the worker hopes that speech will develop with the growth of trust and of a truly human relationship with an adult. Children who seem nonverbal almost always do speak at times, when they are under great stress like the little boy who had the operation, or when they are excited and gay, like one usually mute child who joyfully exclaimed, "Monkey!" as he ran away from the worker. Sometimes speech therapy is recommended. The worker, for his part, must talk frequently to the child, in terms that he can understand, about things that they are doing together. It takes imagination on the worker's part to realize that a youngster may really not understand the meaning of some words that are commonly used and that he may not always know the names of objects. Simple games in which child and worker name and point to various objects are sometimes a great success. As the child gradually becomes able to use language, the worker should not be too ready to accept his nonverbal communications, but should try to get him to ask for what he wants. This rule of course must be used with judgment and not pushed too far.

The first words are likely to be said when the child is with his favorite worker and said in imitation of the worker. This is a critical point in the child's language development, and the worker should make every effort to be available to the child. There have been instances when a worker to whom the child was saying his first words left employment for some reason, and the child stopped talking permanently. This is only one example of the fact that a too rapid turnover of staff is bad for the children. Many treatment centers expect workers to commit themselves to work for at least two years. Temporary workers, perhaps serving during a summer vacation, are cautioned not to relate too deeply to the children.

The child who talks easily and well confronts the worker with an entirely different set of considerations. The worker who is new to his task or is working for the first time with highly verbal children might be tempted to feel that since conversation flows freely, there are no real problems in communication. If he feels this, he will soon be disillusioned. He will need to evaluate his communications to the child, and the child's to him, no less strictly than he does with nonverbal children.

In the first place, he must remember that children in a treatment group are not free to mingle with the neighborhood group of their own age, and that for most of them this separation has been experienced for a long time before they came into treatment, because their behavioral difficulties have cut them off from the peer group. Thus the ordinary exchange of information (and misinformation) that goes on in every neighborhood has not been available to them. They have been unable to adjust their ideas about feelings, things, and people to those of their age-mates. Further, if they are in a residential setting, the workers also substitute for the adults at home who would be expected to answer questions. The children will of necessity turn to the workers (as well as to other children within the treatment group) as a general source of information on many subjects.

Thus much of the conversation that goes on may take the form of questions and answers that enable the children to find out what the world is like—what objects and places are, how they are used, what is dangerous and what is not, but above all how people behave with each other. There will be many questions about the setting of the treatment group in which the children find themselves, often quite personal questions directed to the workers: How many days do you work? What time do you come on duty and when do you go off? Who is your boss, and who is his boss? Who decides whether we can go out and what we will have for lunch? Often the questions refer to the private lives of the workers outside the setting: Where do you live? Do you have a father or a mother, a husband or a wife? (With small children the question, Do you have a father? usually means, Do you have a husband?) Do you have any children? How old are they? Do you ever spank them? Who is the boss at your house, you or your wife? Questions about the setting reflect the real need to know as much as possible about one's own situation, partly for the sake of security, with questions at the back of the child's head, Will I be safe? Will the workers be good to me? Will I always have enough to eat? Will I be abandoned? And this last question, spoken or unspoken, is a very real one.

Sometimes the workers can guess the intent of such questions and can frame their answers to reassure the youngster in his anxiety. In one hospital setting a child had heard that the union of hospital employees had threatened a strike, and he asked anxiously what would happen to the children if none of the workers came in some day. What he wanted was reassurance that someone whom he knew and trusted would be there to care for him, and workers were encouraged to tell him specifically who would be there if a strike occurred. Reassurance could be honestly given since, if a strike had been called, supervisory personnel and non-union workers whom the children knew and were fond of would have worked extra hours to close the gap, just as they would have done in a physical emergency such as a blizzard or a transportation strike. In fact it was possible to tell him just exactly *who* would be there if any emergency arose, and this knowledge was deeply reassuring. The message "We will always take care of you" is one that these anxious children need to hear loudly and clearly, over and over. This type of communication will be discussed later in more detail.

Sometimes questions about the treatment center seem to have the purpose of finding out whom the child can manipulate and how: "If you refuse me a privilege, whom can I go to over your head to get what I want?" When the worker senses such a purpose behind the question, he should let the child know at once in the friendliest way that the worker group is incorruptible (and it must, of course, be incorruptible). The worker may explain that all decisions regarding the children's welfare are made by the staff as a whole and that there is no use in the child's trying to play one against the other. A little gentle kidding is often useful when the youngster is trying to manipulate; maybe he can learn to laugh at himself the next time he tries it.

Questions about the workers' lives outside of the treatment setting also usually come from the children's need for information. They wonder how other people live their lives and how they relate to one another, and it can be very useful for them to get this information. Perhaps a child asks, "Are you the boss at your house, or is your wife the boss?" And the worker replies, "Well, naturally, I decide some things, and she decides some things, and if there is something we don't agree about and we both feel strongly about it, we talk it over and try to come to an agreement." This may be an eye-opener to the child, who may have been exposed to acrimonious arguments between adults or to household tyranny of various kinds. Such an answer, together with his observation that here in the center the workers really do try to work out differences of opinion in a friendly way, may give him an entirely new concept of the way in which people can relate to one another.

The worker will naturally not want to answer every question about his private life, and the decision where to draw the line will depend on many factors, such as the length and quality of his relation with the child, the age and maturity of the child, and his apparent motive in asking the question. He may reply in answer to a child's question, yes, he has girl friends, and he enjoys going out with them; but when the youngster wants to know their names, the worker may very well decline to give them. In reply to questions that workers feel are highly personal, for instance, inquiries about their sex life or about the amount of their salary, workers usually say that that is their private business which they do not usually talk about—though some workers make exceptions even to this, as in Bettelheim's anecdote of the married woman counselor who was asked by a young girl whether she enjoyed intercourse and replied very comfortably that she did.[1]

Beyond a few answers to the children's questions, the worker will not talk to the children about his own family or his own affairs —will not indiscriminately tell him stories of his own children, his own childhood, and the like. Some information-getting questions are likely to be asked, and they are important, but in the main the child needs to think of the worker as a worker, in the milieu in which he and the worker interact. Conversations should be at the child's level, in the here and now of the immediate setting. This is a rule that is usually adhered to very well by the child care workers in settings that are at all sophisticated. What the workers are or what they do outside the treatment center is

1. Bruno Bettelheim, *Love Is Not Enough* (Glencoe, Ill., 1950), pp. 363–64.

not important; what really matters is what they are and what they do at work—how they relate to the children, how they relate to one another.

Aside from personal questions, topics that workers sometimes find difficult to cope with are the general questions of sex, religion, politics, and social issues. The worker's handling of these topics will depend in part on the philosophy of the institution in which he works. For instance, in some centers the questions about sex are referred to the child's individual therapist (e.g., "Why don't you ask Dr. A. about that the next time you see him?"). In some church-related centers religious instruction is part of the regular program. But in most centers a child's questions about any of these emotionally loaded matters are to be answered by the worker simply and factually, without imposing his own biases on the child.

A worker, for instance, who is deeply convinced of the validity of his own creed might feel that it would greatly help a child if he could share his own belief with him. He must realize that it is the prerogative of the parents, not of the worker, to choose whether or not the child shall have religious instruction. He may find himself explaining to the child that there are many different kinds of faith; that among the workers and among the children also there are Catholics, Protestants, and Jews, and some who belong to no church at all; and that the child belongs to a certain church because his parents do; he, the worker, belongs perhaps to a different church, and a third person belongs to still another. A genuinely tolerant attitude on the part of the worker is a great help in a treatment center. The Jewish or the agnostic worker may discover that the little Roman Catholic patient is being prepared for his first Communion, and the child may ask the worker to remind him to say his prayers when he goes to bed or even to help him learn his catechism. Another child may raise tough theological issues that tax the ingenuity of the worker, who may have to say, "I can't really answer that very well because I don't go to the same kind of church you do, but perhaps you could talk to Mrs. B. about it; she goes to your kind of church and I think she would understand."

An impartial, unembarrassed attitude is easier for most workers to achieve in the area of religion than in the area of sex. It takes a certain amount of experience to learn to reply casually to a child who approaches you, for instance, with the question, "Do you have a penis or do you have a vagina?" Yet in all probability he is not trying to insult or embarrass you. He wants to know whether the information he has been given does in fact hold good in all instances, and so he asks. The workers will have to help him understand that there are certain things that can be talked about freely within the center but not outside on the street or in the corner drugstore; within the center his need to know can be satisfied. Transmission of information among workers, and between workers and therapists and supervisory staff, is most important when a child first begins asking questions about any one of the matters that are regarded by adults as "loaded." If the child is having regular visits or is spending his weekends at home, it is important that the parents should know at once what questions he has asked and what answers have been given him in order that they in turn may be able to respond appropriately when he brings the same matters up with them, as he is almost sure to do. The person who communicates with the parents is in most centers the social worker, and it is important that there should be a constant flow of information between the child care workers and the social work staff, so that the parents may be informed of what is going on in the center and the workers conversely may be informed what is going on at home. Only thus can the child be saved much confusion arising from the different handling of many matters.

Communications about death are difficult for many workers to handle, especially when a death has actually occurred in the family of a child or a worker or when a public figure has died. In all such cases honesty rather than concealment should be the rule. If a death has occurred in the immediate family of a worker, it is better that the children should know about it from another worker, who can tell them honestly what has happened and help them with their feelings about it. The worker who has suffered the loss will find it easier if he can stay away from work until he has had an opportunity to cope with his most intense feelings of grief, because the children will almost certainly ask him questions, and although he will want to respond to them honestly, he will want to spare the children a violent outburst of tears on his own part, or the anger that he might feel at their curiosity.

A death in the family of one of the children may present the staff with complicated considerations. The child who has suffered the loss must be told if possible by the adult who is closest to him (his therapist or his own worker) and will need special help from this person over a period of time. This help will be doubly needed if the youngster has any reason to feel especially guilty toward the family member who has died, as happened in one center when the bereaved child had expressed an unusual degree of anger toward her mother for some months before the mother's unexpected and fatal stroke. The worker who helps the child should communicate the substance of their conversations to the rest of the staff so that all can follow through appropriately. Other children who may be especially affected by this child's loss may also need individual consideration; for instance, in the incident cited above, another little girl who had also had unusually angry feelings toward her own mother was extremely upset, asking in panic, "Not *my* mommy?" And then there is the whole group of children, who must be told and who must be helped with their various feelings. If it is decided that the child whose relative has died is to go to the funeral, or to the funeral home, a worker should usually accompany him. When a crisis of this sort arises in a treatment center, the first step is a hasty meeting of all available workers to plan who shall do what for which children, and thereafter communication among workers must be constant so that all aspects of the situation may be handled as well as possible.

The most difficult of all issues to cope with successfully within a treatment setting may often be neither religion or sex or death, but some social issue about which either the workers or the parents feel deeply, such as racial discrimination. Mental health teams in large northern cities have long been integrated, psychiatric understanding being of itself inimical to racial prejudice, and the patient population in any city treatment center is likely to include both white and black children. The ability of the staff members basically to help the children with problems of prejudice depends upon the degree in which they as individuals have been able to overcome their own tendency to be prejudiced and have been able to establish mutual understanding and trust within their own group. At the very least, the decencies must be preserved in any setting hoping to offer treatment. Workers help the children without discrimination; workers are mutually helpful and courteous to one another. To go beyond this sometimes takes hard work, and prejudice is a two-way street. A predominantly Caucasian staff that includes a few Negro members may find its overtly tolerant attitudes undermined by a covert prejudice which workers find it hard to acknowledge and work their way out of. But the writers have also witnessed the opposite phenomenon. An effort was made to balance the worker group on a children's service as regards age, sex, and race by the addition of several young Caucasian male conscientious objectors (who were substituting hospital service for military duty) to a child care staff composed largely of middle-aged, middle-class Negro women. The majority of the workers viewed the newcomers with real suspicion, prepared to find all sorts of peculiarities in them. Experience and discipline, if something less than mutual trust, held the service together at first, until better acquaintance dispelled some of the difficulties.

On the somewhat less touchy subject of political opinions, workers usually find it easy to be frank about their affiliations without trying to proselytize the children. Heated arguments with fellow workers can be deferred until after working hours. One writer remembers the tolerant, slightly amused attitude of seasoned Negro workers toward a schizophrenic teen-ager who had had a cordial exchange of letters with a well-known segregationist politician and was showing the letter that he had received around the center with great pride.

It need hardly be said that the worker should not deceive a child. Within the reasonable limits set by other people's right to privacy, the children have a right to factual answers to their questions. The child's trust in the worker is greatly helped by his realization that the worker's statments can be relied on. The worker may sometimes refuse information if he feels this is necessary, and he may, like anyone else, be mistaken or forget, but he may not deliberately deceive. The child's reliance on the worker is helped, in fact, if the worker can be honest about his own mistakes. He may have promised the children an outing and then have forgotten to make the necessary arrangements, so that the trip has to be cancelled. The easy way out is to tell the children simply, "We can't go," leaving them to assume that some higher power has vetoed the plan. Since the children's self-esteem is low anyway, they are likely to make the assumption that because they are so bad, the pleasure is somehow denied them. If the worker can say honestly, "Gee, I'm terribly sorry, I simply forgot to get the money from the cashier's office before it closed" —or to buy the tickets or the like—the children will know where they stand. They will be angry at the worker and will say so, but relations will be better in the long run. Besides, if the worker has the courage not to allow himself the easy way out, but to face the children's anger, he is less likely to forget the next time, and they are more likely to hold him to his promise. In short, the adult-child relations will be more nearly normal, and this is what treatment is all about.

An aspect of communication which can only be touched on here comes under the heading of "not being fooled by surface behavior or speech." Sometimes what a child says, or what is implied in his behavior, is not his real message. The adult has to look behind the behavior, or behind the words, to discover what the child really means. An example is a youngster who falls and bumps his head hard and comes up smiling or comes up with a perfectly expressionless face. The workers may be deceived into thinking that this child is exceptionally brave when the truth is that he has never learned to turn to an adult for comfort. In chapter 4 an anecdote is told of the boy who was apparently determined not to take his shower in the evenings but was secretly hoping that the workers would show their liking and concern for him by insisting that he take it. Things are not always what they seem. On the other hand, the worker should not fall into the opposite error of never taking the child's communications at face value, of always looking for a second meaning. Disturbed children can at times be perfectly, even devastatingly, honest. If the worker is so fortunate as to have the supervision of a skilled child psychiatrist, he can often receive much help from him in learning to sort out the deceptive communications from the straight ones.

We have been discussing communication between workers and children. We should also note here that constant communication among workers is essential for the best care of the children. This important topic will be discussed in the section on the group of workers in chapter 6.

Response to Feelings

Feelings in disturbed children have not developed in the same way as the feelings of normal children. Disturbed children have to learn to recognize and to distinguish their feelings; workers need to help them with this learning, but to do it with great tact and without intrusiveness. In some children one overwhelming feeling of anxiety seems to be so great that it has drowned out almost all others. In a few even the recognition of anxiety seems to be unbearable, and they have retreated into extreme withdrawal. After the worker gets acquainted with disturbed children for the first time and begins to see behind their peculiar behavior and to understand why this one perpetually plays with a piece of string, that one walks and talks rather like a robot, a third dashes breathlessly from one toy to the other never stopping to play with anything, and a fourth hits out at other children without seeming reason, he will slowly become aware of their pervasive anxiety, or better said, their *lack of trust*. The least trustful children do not seem actually to feel anxiety; they simply withdraw into themselves. It is only after they have developed a relationship with someone, and have a little experience of trust,

that they seem also to be able to encounter anxiety as a feeling—
to reexperience the anxiety that they have avoided by withdrawing. Less withdrawn children who attack other children or who
suddenly scratch and bite a worker without seeming provocation
are also responding to anxiety or to the lack of trust but in another
way, as are the children who run away, set fires, or steal, and
even those who bully others and try to manipulate adults.

The worker thus learns to look for anxiety behind the compulsive playing with string of one child, behind the continual slap-
ping of himself of a second, behind the mechanical behavior of
a third, and behind the "misbehavior" of a fourth. These are
frightened children, but, equally, anxiety is so much a part of
their lives that they often do not realize that they are anxious.
Sometimes they can recognize their fears, and talk about them,
only after they have partially overcome them. The worker must
realize that such anxieties can be overcome only slowly, as the
child gains trust in the world around him and also in his own
powers. What the worker can do about them is to notice the times
when the child seems particularly anxious—when he withdraws
more, or is more restless, or attacks, or simply displays fears of
certain objects or people—and then to reassure him that he will
be safe, that the workers will care for him.

In one group the children were taken on frequent hikes during the
summer. When they came to a place in the woods where there were
huge, overhanging rocks on both sides of the trail, one of the children,
an eight-year-old, would try to run away, would begin to laugh in a
high-pitched, nonhumorous way, and obviously would be feeling very
upset. The worker would simply reassure him that he was safe, since
she really did not know what was upsetting him. (Was it the relative
darkness because of so many trees, or the trees themselves, or being
so far away from school, or the creek near by?) Two years later, on
the same path, the youngster said, "I thought those rocks were going
to fall on me, and they're still there."

Some of the obvious periods of anxiety are times of separation,
for example, when a child is admitted to or discharged from a
treatment center, in a lesser degree when children in residential

treatment say good-by to their parents after a visit, when those in day care leave their parents in the morning, or when a worker whom the children are dependent on goes off duty. At such times a worker can help the child with his feelings. This help can often take the form of *response to the feeling*, rather than statements *about* the feeling. In the case of the newly admitted child, one worker is usually assigned to show him around, introduce him to children and workers, assure him that he will be cared for and that it is natural to be scared in a new place and to miss his mother and father. Other separation pangs, for example, after visits, can be dealt with similarly. The worker going off duty can tell the children when he will be on duty again, and he may also say who will care for them in the meantime and reiterate that they will be safe. Even when a worker whom the children are accustomed to depending on has to leave the group temporarily for some reason, he may find it wise to tell them as he leaves when he will be back and who will care for them while he is gone. Similarly, the substitute worker, if he notes signs of unusual anxiety among the children during the absence of their regular worker, can assure them that their worker is only away for a time, that he will be back, and if possible just when to expect him. In addition, the absence of one of the children from the group can in itself make the others anxious and should be explained to them.

The writers can recall one totally nonverbal eight-year-old child, sitting with other children at a table for a "meeting" and pointing to each of the others over and over until one of the adults recognized that he was missing one of his mates. When he was told, "Sammy is all right. He is a little upset, and Sarah is talking to him in the other room," he stopped pointing and attended to the business of the meeting.

It is good practice to state habitually to the group why a child is out of the room, what is happening (he is safe), and when he will be back. If a child is absent from a day care group for a day or several days, it is important to remember to tell the children why he is away (he isn't feeling well, he is resting, his mother is taking good care of him) and when he will be back. Permanent departure of anyone from the group, worker or child, needs careful preparation. If a worker is leaving, it is desirable if possible that the children meet their new worker before the old one has left and that they be assured many times over that the new worker will take good care of them just as the former worker has done. And the departing worker should be prepared for some punishment at the hands of the children. They will almost certainly act up or regress during his last days of duty. It is good if the former worker can come back for a visit or two, so that the children will not have the fantasy that people die or simply disappear when they leave the group. When a child is being discharged from the group, the other children should know where and why he is going—"He is better now and is going to a regular school" or perhaps "He is going to a different center where people will help him." Often when a worker or a child is leaving, a good-by party is part of the ceremony.

There is usually anxiety for a child in residential treatment *before* a visit from his parents or a trip home, presumably in the fear that unless his behavior is acceptable, the parents may not come again or may not take him home again.

One nine-year-old in residential treatment regularly had a violent temper tantrum on Friday nights before his scheduled home visits on Saturday. A worker in his group, who knew the child very well, used to say, while holding him during his tantrums and preventing him from biting himself or her and from hitting his head against the wall, "All right, Bobby, all right. You're going home tomorrow, and I think that's why you're so excited tonight." After some months of this, Bobby began to say spontaneously on Friday nights: "I know. Bessie [the worker] would say, 'Bobby, you're excited because you're going home tomorrow.'" And as he became able to identify his own feelings, the tantrums diminished and finally stopped.

Statements *about* the child's feelings are not always to be avoided but should only be made when the youngster has given clear cues to the worker and then, at first, tentatively: "Maybe you were a

little bit scared." It does no good for the worker to try to identify
the precise feeling that the child has unless the child can recognize the same feeling.

Any change, any new experience, makes the children anxious.
If the group is to undertake a new activity or to go to a new
place, it is essential to tell the children ahead of time where they
are going and what they will do. It is essential also to talk about
the rules of behavior at that particular place: people do not pick
flowers at the conservatory; they must stay behind the railing at
the zoo, and so on. And, as always, the workers must emphasize
that the children will be safe. When they come to a place where
the surroundings are strange, the workers can explain what it is
they are seeing, and again after the trip they can talk about what
they have seen and done and prepare them for doing it again
some day. In this discussion the workers should include some of
the children's feelings about the experience, helping them to
express these if they can but in any case making some general
statements: "Children often feel a little bit scared in a new place"
and perhaps adding, "But it was fun, wasn't it?"—if it clearly was.
The world seems so chaotic to disturbed children that they really
often do not understand ordinary things that other children would
take in stride. A senior staff member in a treatment center, giving
directions to a volunteer who was to take a little girl, relatively
new to the center, out in her car to buy her own birthday cake,
said something like the following: "Tell her everything that is
happening as you go: 'Now we are stopping for a red light.' 'Now
I am parking the car,' and so forth, for the whole trip." The trip
was highly successful. The worker's object is not to shield the
children from all anxiety but to expose them to small, bearable
amounts of it by gradually giving them experiences that other
children have, to the extent that they can accept them, and in
the process help them to cope with the anxiety that is an unavoid-
able part of experience. Such planning provides, as one worker
said, "the deliberately programmed necessity for them to trust."
The little girl would not have been sent on the trip at all if the

object had been to shield her from all anxiety. Putting her into the car with the volunteer provided the "programmed necessity for her to trust," but the careful instructions to the volunteer made the anxiety "a small, bearable amount" by making it possible for the child to master the experience, piece by piece, through understanding.

Mingled with the anxiety, or, perhaps better said, a component of it, seems to be the disturbed child's frequent concept of himself as bad, deficient, or somehow not entirely human. Children who can play out their fantasies frequently represent themselves in their games by such figures as the bad baby or the robot. One child, whose play is described elsewhere in this chapter, said, "At home I'm the Tin Man, and at school I'm the Cowardly Lion." Children who do not play sometimes enact the same feeling in their behavior, for example, the children who hit themselves or the little nonverbal boy who, holding a toy dog, pressed his thumbs against the dog's glass eyes and then hid his face as if in shame (he had been punished at the age of two for trying to gouge his baby brother's eyes). When disturbed children in an elementary learning situation comply for the first time with what the worker asks of them, they often do so in a seemingly shame-faced, backhanded manner—sometimes with a quick gesture and an equally quick withdrawing of the hand. This attitude is often described as stubbornness, but to the observer on the sidelines it seems as if the child were telegraphing, "I'm a bad, nonlearning boy. I really shouldn't be doing what you ask me to, but I'll do it just this once and hope nobody will really see me do it." To this kind of feeling the worker can only reply by letting the child know that he *is* valued—he and everything about him, his possessions, his achievement. Every achievement should be met with warm encouragement, but extravagant praise will be too much for the child and he may go out of his way not to achieve the next time.

Anger in a disturbed child is so much a part of anxiety that it is hard to disentangle the two feelings, but if the experience that the child is reacting to is one in which he might appropriately be angry—as when he has been attacked by another child—it is important to help him realize this feeling. It is important to help him direct his anger to the right person: "It's not me you're angry at. It was Tommy who hit you. You can let him know you're angry." In a withdrawn child angry behavior is often a real gain; it means that he is at last able to release some of the feelings that he has been holding in behind his facade of withdrawal. As was said earlier, it is important not to force him to turn his aggression back on himself. This point needs emphasis, because inexperienced workers are likely to feel that a child who suddenly becomes aggressive and difficult is "worse." In many cases it is the child's first step toward health, and if the worker is observant, he may notice that the same child is making little advances in his positive relation to people at the same time; for instance he may put his arms around the worker when he has never done so before.

A child's first angry behavior may take deplorable forms. Because he is angry at the biggest and strongest child in the room, he may turn on the smallest and weakest and try to beat him up. Workers have to know how to restrain him without damaging his ability to get appropriately angry the next time. He has a right to his anger, and if his earliest efforts to express it are not those of a good Boy Scout, we should hardly be surprised. Likely as not, the first target of his anger will be the worker—in the long process of teasing and defying that workers refer to as "testing." The worker is the safest target, because the child knows he will not retaliate. For months on end, the child may continue to do the things that he knows will bother the worker the most: he may dawdle with dressing, wet the floor just after the worker has taken him to the bathroom, or tear up other children's artwork. He seems to be fulfilling the double need of expressing his pent-up anger and assuring himself that the workers will still accept him no matter how bad he is. Workers can shorten this process if they recognize the feeling and talk about it to the child.

In the case of aggressive interaction between children, the worker must of course not let any child get hurt. Differences among children can sometimes be safely and socially structured into competitive sports. Physically abusive behavior can sometimes be directed to things that can take it, for example, knockdown toys, woodwork, the sandbox, depending on the age and competence of the given child. With an active, domineering child, a bully, isolation from the other children is sometimes necessary, but the temptation is to use isolation too much, and the worker can usefully look for alternatives. It helps to point out to the bully just what he is doing and also to point out to the other children, his victims, that they are part of his bullying. They can be encouraged to say to him, "I don't like to do that" or "I'm not going to play with you if you do that." This social isolation may bring the bully into a subdued frame of mind in which he may be much more reachable than he was before.

Jealousy is an important cause of anger, especially when a child is just coming to be fond of certain workers and wants their full attention.

One nonverbal six-year-old would sit on the laps of workers he liked, but if another child approached, he would get up as if he had lost interest and go off to another part of the room. It would have been easy to miss the feeling behind this behavior, and it is possible that the child himself was hardly aware of the feeling at first. This youngster had for a long time not been able to accept closeness from anybody. Then he seemed to awaken to the presence of caring adults in his environment, and he would come out of periods of withdrawal and hug the workers around the neck with smiles and squeals of delight, much like those of a small baby. He was given much undivided adult attention, but there were necessarily times when the workers had to care for other children too. His gesture of going away when another child approached the worker seemed to express his fear that if the worker paid attention to another child he himself would be totally abandoned. He had ultimately to learn that a worker could like and take care of more than one child at a time but that in spite of this fact his needs would always be met and he would always be cared for. Workers said to him: "It seems to me that every time Jimmy comes to me for help, you go away. Maybe you're afraid I don't like you when I help Jimmy. I can like and take care of you and Jimmy and Sara and Tony and Jean [other children in the group]" or sometimes simply, "I like you even when I'm helping Jimmy."

Another child in a different group, perhaps feeling a similar terror that she might be abandoned in favor of the other children and a need to have for herself all the love of both the adults who cared for the group, attacked the other children in the group indiscriminately. She was restrained and reassured, and very gradually began to accept the fact that the adults could care for her and the others too.

Anxiety and anger are the most conspicuous feelings that the children are likely to express, but positive feelings are there too. The most important of these is the children's dependence on, and identification with, the child care workers. It is a revelation to a new worker to realize how important he becomes to the children and how some of them identify with him and unconsciously or consciously imitate him, and to realize also that the way in which he responds to them is very important to them and that they also notice and are influenced by the way in which he responds to other children and to other staff members. It is not unusual to see a child imitate the gait and speech of one of the workers.

One aggressive, hyperactive boy in a day care center was unable to get a haircut because when the barber approached his hair with the scissors he became so anxious that he would throw bottles and other glass around. His child care worker one day took the boy to the barber shop with him while he himself got a haircut. Two days later the boy showed up with a haircut, proudly proclaiming, "I get a haircut; I be like John; I sit quiet."

This emotional reliance of the child on the worker is most important and must be recognized and respected. *Good relationships with the adults that are available to him in the treatment center are the chief means by which the child gets better.* The adults on their part must be what one worker calls "emotionally available," open and receptive to what the children bring to them.

Sooner or later a child in a treatment group also begins to relate to other children, though his relatedness may show itself more obliquely than it does in a group of normal children, for example, in anxiety when another child is temporarily away from the group. Children are aware of the other children, but overt interaction is subtle. Often the first interaction that occurs among withdrawn children takes the form of avoidance or of imitation and is almost invisible unless one is watching closely. Two withdrawn children may be occupying opposite corners of the playroom; one gets up and wanders toward the opposite corner; the second gets up and wanders toward the corner which the first occupied. They have not been close to each other, yet they have been aware of each other—they have changed places. Or one child will lie down on the floor and lay his head on the foot of a child care worker; on the other side of the room another child will lie down and lay *his* head on the foot of a different worker. The two actions do not seem related, yet they have occurred one after the other. And all workers soon realize that withdrawn children imitate each other's symptomatic behavior. Direct interaction with an overtone of "fun" often begins when one child playfully hits another and runs away, looking back and laughing as if expecting to be chased. When the children are less withdrawn, the interaction is easier to observe. A given child may be hostile and aggressive or may try to manipulate others to fill his own needs. The less disturbed children will be able to play together after the fashion of other children, but it is usually a long time before severely disturbed children can play with one another in the manner of ordinary children. For this reason it is better not to have a whole group of withdrawn children but to include verbal with nonverbal children, active with passive ones. The active children initiate interaction, so the withdrawn children are more quickly drawn into it. Ultimately certain children show awareness of the needs of other children; one of them may tell a worker that so-and-so is upset and needs help. Signs of relatedness and signs of enjoyment on the part of the children are closely watched for and quickly responded to by the workers, and programming is planned to promote opportunities for children to interact with one another.

It is important for the workers to recognize and encourage any friendships among the children. Workers can take account of these friendships in grouping, planning for trips, and so on.

Friendships are signs of health and as such warrant careful discussion in staff meetings. Sometimes the attachment of two children may take a problematical form; for instance, one child may continually offer himself to be tormented, and the other may seem to want to torment him, both trying to outwit the workers in what seems a highly perverse activity; or a bigger child may constantly try to involve a smaller one in sex play, and the smaller one may enjoy it enough to cooperate. No blanket rule covers all cases, and much discussion is necessary. Often better program planning so that there are more things for the children to do that they enjoy doing will make it possible to preserve the relationship between the children while the undesirable behavior drops out. Disturbed children rarely see themselves as sources of pleasure to other people, that is, they rarely give gratification to others without exacting a heavy price. The concept that individuals can simply enjoy each other ("We liked the lions and the lions liked us," as one child put it) dawns slowly. It is important, therefore, when one child obviously enjoys another, to help him to appreciate that he can be enjoyed in his turn.

Disturbed children seldom really seem to have fun in any activity, and workers are always looking for ways to awaken the feeling of enjoyment in them. The first realization by a child that he is "having fun" marks a real step toward health. Very withdrawn small children often show their first enjoyment at kinesthetic pleasure—at being tossed up or whirled around. This activity is all right as a way to help them begin to relate to adults; it should not go on month after month, however, but should be replaced by forms of play in which the child himself participates. (And be aware that tickling is usually too stimulating for a disturbed child, even if he seems to ask for it. There are plenty of other ways to help him get acquainted with his body.) Other forms of play, involving mastery—like going down a slide, manipulating a toy, or putting together a puzzle or a model—may rouse a feeling of anxiety at first when they are new and untried and then pleasure and even real joy when they are mastered. All these feelings are the worker's concern, and in a sense he participates in them with the child, helping the child to make them real to himself.

Throughout the day's activities the workers are thus continually recognizing and responding to the children's feelings, either verbally or nonverbally, but always simply and with tact and honesty. The child must be aware that the worker knows how he feels and that he understands. Much of the art of child care work lies in the timing, appropriateness, and manner of these expressions of feeling. Clumsy and too pointed references to feelings may make the child withdraw and may prevent expression next time. Above all, the worker who needs to make the child feel that he has "got the goods on him" has missed his calling. He should be in some other line of business. Warm, brief, sympathetic (and occasionally humorous) responses from the adult's feeling to the child's feeling make the child aware that he is understood and respected, make his feeling more real to him, and make him more able to act on his feeling when that is appropriate or to take care of it in some other way. Every good child care worker develops his own style of responding to feeling. This is one of those things that essentially cannot be learned from books. The student needs to watch experienced child care workers in action, to try out his own skills with the children under their supervision, and to have ample opportunity afterward to discuss the nuances of interaction with his supervisors. One good rule of thumb is to use simple language when talking with children. The worker may have read a great deal of child psychology and may know a great many technical terms, but all concepts should be translated into simple everyday language for the child's benefit. Worries, for instance, is a better term to use with children than anxieties.

Expectations and Limit-setting

Whether they work with withdrawn children or with children with behavior disturbances, child care workers have certain expectations for change and growth on the part of the children. The worker who is in charge of withdrawn, out-of-contact children encourages and expects each child to perform tasks that are closer and closer to those which children of his age usually perform. He looks for what is healthy in the child, for what he *can* do, and builds on that. Before he can do this, the worker may first have to interfere at times with symptomatic behavior that is occupying most of the child's energy. For instance, to take four examples from one group of disturbed children, one child is occupied in continually twisting string; one divides his time between drawing circles around the numbers of pages in books and hunting around the floor to pick up pieces of lint and paper; one wants to engage the workers in a repetitious conversation that prevents his doing anything else; one wants to spend the day opening and shutting doors in a particular way.

Among treatment centers which have made real progress in the treatment of severely disturbed children, practice differs somewhat as to the manner and duration of these interruptions of symptomatic behavior, but there is agreement that if the child is to make any progress at all, there must be some "teaching" in the elementary sense of that word. The director of one center interferes with symptomatic behavior at first "only for a split second" to get the child to do something at the adult's request which he may soon learn to enjoy doing for its own sake. This is followed up on successive days with gentle persistence till the participation in the adult-initiated activity becomes a source of pleasure to the child, and the adult's approval serves as a reward. Every effort is made by the adult to follow the child's clues in suggesting activities, and any flicker of interest is followed up. In another center the adults present a simple activity and expect that the child will do something with it, however little at first. For instance, small blocks are put out on the table; the children are expected to sit together at the table and handle the blocks in some way—touch them, smell them, roll them around. They need not attempt to build anything at first unless they wish. The adults persist in their expectation in the face of anxiety "expressed often with tantrums, tears, shouting, and attempts to bite or kick the worker."

With all their kindly firmness, however, the workers in neither center punish the children for their reluctance to participate. What the worker attempts to reproduce in these expectations of performance is the interaction between a mother and a very young child who is learning to manipulate objects through play. Somehow in the lives of these children this interaction has not taken place and the learning has been bypassed. An observer who sees a skilled worker going through this process with a disturbed child is struck by the fact that at first this is not a particularly happy interaction for the child and that his gestures, if he does what the adult asks him to, often suggest shame or self-doubt. He half wants to please the adult and is half embarrassed to. As we noted earlier, his self-concept seems to be that he is a person who does *not* comply, is *not* competent, and does *not* please; but every little success, every little pleasure at the adult's approval, helps him in some small measure to change his self-concept.

Some workers have been able to relate to severely disturbed children by joining their repetitive activity and then gradually changing the pattern, saying something like, "I'm going to do it differently. Can you do it differently too?" Such an approach has to be made carefully, since the child may view the choice of activity as too destructive. He is likely in any case to be somewhat upset. But trust is enhanced when such an effort succeeds, as it did in the case of one youngster who perpetually clapped his hands. The worker joined the handclapping and after some time varied the rhythm and the child followed. Then the child varied the rhythm (with a big grin) and the adult followed. In this way the first communication was set up.

Ultimately, the child's own sense of mastery, the satisfaction of his strivings for autonomy, will be the real reward and the real spur to further learning. Along the way the small rewards in his interaction with the adult—the adult's commendations, the success in some small thing, the pleasure of imitating the adult—are what keep him going. These little rewards are some of the means by which every small child learns. Helping a child to undertake and ultimately to have satisfaction in a task that he has hitherto avoided requires slow, steady, patient effort and a sensitivity to the child's changing responses.

Bill, a nonverbal seven-year-old, had never helped himself in any way; his hands were flaccid and he had gradually to develop the use of them. The workers undertook to help him learn to put his boots on when he was going outdoors. The first emphasis was on the idea, "It's all right to ask for help," and on the effort to get him to indicate what he wanted. First they had to be sure that he knew what the words *locker* and *boots* meant. When they said to him, "Go to your locker and get your boots" and he did so, they considered this evidence that he *did* know what the words meant. Gradually, by asking him, "Do you want something?" the workers got him to say, "Boots." The next step, carefully timed, was to get him to "try." At first he would make just one little gesture; then he slowly reached the point where he would really struggle to put the boots on—on most days, that is. After a hard day the workers felt this requirement was too much, and on such days they would help him. Discovering that being tired brought help, he sometimes tried to enact fatigue, but his worker, with a sharp eye for pretense, would say, "Nice try, Bill, but I know you're kidding," at which he would smile broadly. She invented a "boot song" when he began to do up the buckles. "First you buckle, buckle number one; then you buckle, buckle number two; then you buckle, buckle number three; then you shift to the other boot." As he progressed in this, for him, really difficult task, Bill's satisfaction was intense.

An experienced worker can often tell intuitively when a child is ready to give up an immature or disturbed form of behavior and proceed to another level.

Peter spent much time in the repetitive activity of circling numbers in books and magazines. No effort was made until he was far advanced on his way to health to get him to give up this activity entirely, though it was interfered with periodically and progressively from the beginning when he was asked to take part in other activities. Finally, about a year and a half after he had entered the treatment center (he was now ten), the worker sensed that he was ready to give up this activity but needed to be helped to do so. She said to him, "After vacation, no more Wall-Tex." (He was using a book of wallpaper samples for his circling.) He said simply, "Okay." After vacation he asked for his wallpaper book, but when he was reminded that he was to give it up after vacation, he simply grinned. He went on asking for a few days but seemed relieved when it was refused. He had really been ready, with a little help, to give it up. Now he started a round of new activities. He appropriated all the toy animals, painting them, washing them off, dumping the water (sometimes on the floor), throwing things, instigating others to throw. At the same time he began to work on differentiation of feelings: "What does *sad* mean? *mad? glad?*" He appropriated adults to write lists for him, for instance, lists of feelings. Concurrently, he started to make progress in the classroom.

Planning with the expectation of growth on the part of a whole group will take into account the children's capacities, needs, and anxieties and can offer a graduated series of challenges and satisfactions.

An illustration of this is the planning in a day treatment center for young severely disturbed children for a series of trips. The first venture involved simply walks around the neighborhood, with an adult holding each child's hand, and emphasis on coming back always to the familiar and safe premises of the center. Extending the walks a little farther, the group began to visit a playground a few blocks away, where bigger and more varied apparatus was available than at the center and which thus offered greater challenges and more varied kinds of pleasure. A few blocks away in another direction were some stores, and the children were taken to some of these, for instance to choose the kind of cookies they would buy. On all these trips the first emphasis, spoken or implied, was on the idea, "You are safe, we will take care of you, and at the end of the trip we all will get back safely to the center." Once the children had begun to incorporate this feeling, the emphasis (again not always spoken but always implied in the tone and behavior of the workers) was not only that "this is fun," but also that there are ways of behaving toward other people. For instance, on walks people do not like to be yelled at and at the bakery, "We will buy the cookies you want, but we can't let you grab them."

After trips around the neighborhood had become successful and pleasurable to the children, the group undertook several trips to the zoo, with careful preparation beforehand. The workers were aware that many children are somewhat afraid of animals, partly because to them they represent the impulsiveness, perhaps the oral aggression, that they themselves have only partially conquered. For the same reason, if the fear can be overcome, the animals are particularly fascinating to the children. After the children had begun to enjoy the zoo, trips were taken to a natural history museum, where the children saw, among other things, some stuffed animals. The workers were alert for the ideas and feelings that might arise here around the fact that the animals are dead ("How did they get that way?"), that they are stuffed ("Who stuffs them? Do the animals mind it?") etc. These trips cannot be a one-shot deal. It was important to go back again and again to these fear-arousing places, so that the children, little by little, could master the tremendous anxiety engendered.

Much later, when the children had gained still more security, the group went to a circus, where they saw animals with no bars between them and their trainers, and this too they were able to master and enjoy. To one little girl the circus was so important an experience that she asked to go again. She wanted her parents to take her, but for extra security she wanted the worker with whom she had gone the first time to come along too, and this was arranged.

This sequence of activities is only one among many possible illustrations of the sharpened awareness that workers need to have when they plan learning experiences for the children.

As we noted in the discussion of anger, when a withdrawn child comes out of his shell, his behavior often appears to be worse, and it may be necessary, provisionally, for the worker to accept behavior that he will later expect the child to modify and for the child to understand that the worker does accept it only provisionally. As one worker of long experience puts it, "Something is operating in me that accepts—doesn't inhibit—but doesn't really condone." To the child she says, "I don't really like it, but if you need to do it I'll accept it for now." Most withdrawn children who improve become temporarily "acter-outers." It seems as though their withdrawal had protected them against their own impulses, and when the workers have coaxed them out of this withdrawal, some of the unacceptable impulses begin to be acted on and such things as temper tantrums and expressions of anger begin to show themselves. The worker should not make the mistake of thinking that the child is worse. To a certain extent he must accept the child's expressions of anger, but it is also his task to help the child out of this temporary state—to sense when the youngster is able to give up this kind of behavior and to help him on to the next stage of more acceptable conduct.

Reliance on a rigid and especially on an extreme system of

rewards and punishments is to be avoided by all means in work with withdrawn children. It can indeed occasionally produce results. In an extremity of anxiety, the children may become compliant to the adults, but their compliance is not to be construed as improvement. The writers have seen such a result produced by the mother of a nine-year-old withdrawn boy, who carried a switch with her at all times when she was with the child. He could not talk or play, but he followed her directions like a little robot. Real mastery of appropriate tasks, on the other hand, allows children to feel better about themselves, gains recognition from the people around them, and helps them gradually to approach the society of other boys and girls from which some of them have been alienated and in which some have never participated.

The purpose of discipline is, after all, to enable the child to internalize the controls which the child care worker must temporarily furnish. If a child's behavior is too much for the others in the group to take, the usual procedure in good treatment centers is to take him into another room, where the worker stays with him and talks to him—talks *with* him, if the child can talk—about the feelings that may have brought on the behavior. The reader should remember what was said earlier about the "tentative approach." A skilled worker does not attribute feelings to the child but merely suggests what they may be.[2] Sometimes it is necessary for the worker to hold a child firmly to prevent him from hurting himself or the worker; there will be more about this later.

In the case of verbal and more competent children, in whom behavior problems are often conspicuous, the expectations of the worker center in ego control, not in initial learning. Such children are not prevented from taking part in ordinary children's activi-

2. Staying with a child is a good general rule, but there are times when it is wiser for the worker to leave the child alone in the room and wait outside, for instance, if the child really seems to need time alone to pull himself together or in the occasional instance when a disturbed boy is sexually excited by the presence of a woman worker and no male worker is available.

ties such as school, games, and daily tasks; but their performance may be impeded or interrupted by their emotional problems, as their satisfaction in their own achievement often is. For instance, a boy may make a number of model airplanes over a period of weeks and display them in his room with apparent pride, but he suddenly destroys them all in a fit of despondency. Behavior that prevents a child from fully participating in and enjoying the program often seems like that of a much younger child—wanting all the materials for himself, sulking if some other child is assisted before he is, disrupting other people's work. Most disconcerting to the worker may be his tendency to fly off the handle and to resort to violent or destructive behavior. Children may fight, bully other children, break up equipment, and otherwise create chaos. With such children the expectations on the part of the worker will nevertheless be closer to those which he would have for a normal child than for the very withdrawn child. Staff discussions must center on just what safeguards this child needs, what allowances must be made, and what step ahead he is ready for.

The principles which the worker needs to keep in mind in dealing with these less withdrawn but still very difficult children are basically the same as with the more withdrawn, but there are differences of application.[3] In order for the children to improve, the workers must really be able to stop them, if need be, from hurting themselves or each other, from breaking up property, disrupting the program, or doing anything else that will result in too great anxiety or guilt. The young normal child, when he is building up his ego-capacities and controls, counts on the adult to function provisonally as his ego—to do those things for him that he cannot yet do for himself and to protect him from his own impulses by preventing him from doing things that would injure him or other people or have other adverse effects. The child with

---

3. There are fortunately some guides already published for workers with such children. See Albert E. Trieschman, James K. Whittaker, and Larry K. Brendtro, *The Other Twenty-three Hours* (Chicago, 1969) and the older classic, Fritz Redl and David Wineman, *The Aggressive Child* (Glencoe, Ill., 1957). Both are written on a more advanced level than this volume.

a behavior problem is one in whom, for whatever reason, this development has not fully taken place. Some of the testing of the worker that children with behavior problems do early in their relations with him (and that withdrawn children eventually do if they get better) seems to have the purpose of finding out whether the adult is strong enough to afford the kind of control that is needed. (Teachers, baby-sitters, and other adults also are tested by the children in their charge, though usually in a milder way.) An experienced worker can often meet the defiance of a child (perhaps with a little gentle humor) so that it melts away, but fundamentally all the children must understand that the workers will protect them from external and internal aggression. No child can be allowed to hurt himself, another child, or the worker; nor can destruction of property on any appreciable scale be permitted. Once the children understand this—and they often have to test many times before they believe it—a long step toward trust has been taken.

For this kind of security to be real, there must be enough workers to control the children, and they must be vigilant enough to do so. When intervention does become necessary, workers must be able to control their charges without hurting them. The child care staff should have the opportunity to talk together with an experienced child care worker or psychiatric nurse about ways of restraining a child without making it too painful or "taking it out" on him. Workers must avoid the too sharp yank on the arm, the too tight and painful grip. The adult must be aware of his own anger, which may be aroused by the physical effort and by the child's defiance, and must not be seduced into punishing the child by hanging on to him in a way that hurts. There are ways of holding that provide warm security and control at the same time, and this is true even if the child to be held is quite big and several adults are necessary.

One of the writers recalls a delinquent adolescent who went berserk in his apparent need to test the new male director of a day-care unit. It required four men—the director, two counselors, and a student—to hold him for nearly an hour while the director talked reassuringly to him. The boy was big and very strong. The number of men made it possible to control him without hurting him and also, the director felt, saved his pride. There was no shame in being controlled by several men, whereas to be caught in some special hold by one counselor would have been humiliating as well as painful. After that incident it was over; he had tested the director, had been controlled, and had not been hurt. The boy had never done such a thing before (at least at the center), and he did not do it again.

With skillful child care work the need for physical control is minimized, but it must be available if needed.

Even in purely verbal interchange it is sometimes hard to remember to respond therapeutically, rather than punitively or moralistically, to a child who has tried the worker's patience. There is a temptation to say, "I'm surprised you can ask a favor of me this afternoon after the way you behaved this morning," when the worker really should have noted the anxiety behind the outburst of the morning and already should have responded in some way to it. This is not to say that these particular words, from worker to child, are a mistake in all instances. There might be times, if they were said with warmth, when they would be exactly right as conveying the worker's truly justified exasperation. But they are overused. The better response in most instances would be, "Look, Bill, you seemed pretty upset this morning after your visit last night. Do you think you are able to go to the store this afternoon?" There are, of course, plenty of times when a worker becomes unavoidably angry. This point is discussed further in the section on the worker's feelings in chapter 6.

It is a sound rule that one should talk with a child as soon as possible about something that has caused upset behavior on his part, since the feelings that have accompanied the upset are often very fleeting, especially with action-oriented children, and he may quite honestly not be able to remember later on why he behaved as he did. Soon after the event a child who has a good relationship with the worker may be able to tell him something of what it was that made him "fly off the handle." His appointment with his therapist may have been suddenly cancelled or something the worker did may have been construed as favoritism to another child; and when the feeling that prompted the behavior is still fresh, he may be able to tell the worker what it was and thus make some real progress.[4] But this technique, like any other, has to be used with discrimination. If it is pursued day after day, the chances are that the child really does not know what is upsetting him, but since the worker expects an explanation, he gives him one off the top of his head: "So-and-so made me angry," or the like. Close observation of the child's play will often be more fruitful, as in some of the situations described in chapter 5.

Although the problem of limiting aggression is ubiquitous in treatment centers, whatever their size, the problem of limiting sex play appears to be less perplexing in the small center where there are plenty of workers and where psychiatric guidance is readily available. A new worker confronted for the first time with sex exploration or play between a boy and a girl or between two children of the same sex, or with open masturbation on the part of a young child may find that his first reaction is hysterical or punitive.[5] He may be rather surprised to find that his supervisors take these things rather calmly. In his effort to adopt their non-punitiveness, he may swing over to the opposite attitude, interpreting *nonpunitiveness* to mean that in this place anything goes, that behavior that would be unacceptable in the community at large can be indulged in freely behind the walls of a treatment center. The children, who are only doing, perhaps with less discretion and self-control, the same things that children have always done, are thus caught in the middle. If the workers respond punitively, the children, who already have little enough self-esteem, will be made to feel that they are even more worth-

4. See Fritz Redl, "Strategy and Techniques of the Life Space Interview," *American Journal of Orthopsychiatry* 29 (January 1958), pp. 1–18.

5. For a fuller discussion of handling sex problems, the reader is referred to p. 158 in chapter 9. That passage represents the combined thinking of several authors and can be applied as well in the small center as in the large institution.

less. On the other hand, if the workers abdicate their responsibility and allow the children to do things which they, the workers, know would not be permitted by society outside of a special environment, they fail the children in a very crucial area. The goal is to return the children, if possible, to the community or, even if they remain institutionalized, to permit them to go outside the institution for trips and special events, not to shut them up inside the buildings at all times. As in any limit-setting, we are concerned to intervene therapeutically in order to help the child build up his inner controls, to substitute acceptable activity for what is unacceptable, and to do it in a way that will enhance his relations with other people and that will not lower his self-esteem. The worker should be reminded here that exploration involves the need to know and that while we are here concerned with limit-setting, communication is part of the same package.

The worker's approval is important to a child who is struggling for better controls and is one incentive for him to work on his problems. Being aware of this, the worker should not withhold his recognition of the child's achievement. On the other hand, he should not urge or imply, "Do it for me." The child grows and achieves for his own sake. For the more competent, verbal child, some tangible recognition may be meaningful, whether it be candy, a privilege, a special treat, or the tokens or points of the more formal reward systems—something more symbolic, in other words, than just the approval of the worker. In working with the younger child, who needs *rearing* rather than *treatment,* the worker can count on himself as a very important person, and his response, along with the child's own sense of mastery, is often reward enough. A child who is competent in self-care and in other things needs the worker less, and though for him too the worker's approval and the sense of achievement are important, a tangible reward is often a great incentive.

Punishment can occasionally be useful for a child who is competent enough to have some control of his behavior and to recognize that he is deliberately misbehaving, assuming, again, that the worker who punishes already has a good relationship with him.

In one day center a ten-year-old youngster who had improved greatly and was almost ready for public school became angry and broke a window. Because the workers were sure that he really could have controlled his anger and could have expressed it in some more acceptable way, he was sent home for the rest of the day and was required to pay for the repair of the window out of his allowance. Earlier in his treatment, when his self-control had not been established, he would simply have been restrained from further damage and an effort made to find out what was upsetting him.

Punishment that is applied in such a situation, with warmth and understanding, is not felt by the child as hostile. It says to him, "I know that you can control your behavior, and I like you enough to risk distressing you a little to help you with it." This sort of punishment requires the child to make compensation for a destructive act. In different circumstances, such compensation might require not the payment of money but some effort on the child's part—cleaning up a mess he has made, repairing something he has broken.

Temporary separation from the group when a child is disruptive and when in the worker's judgment he is really capable of controlling himself but is not trying hard enough can be used as punishment and is felt by the child as such, especially when some pleasurable activity is under way. This separation is different from taking a child who really cannot control himself away from the group in order to help him gain composure. If the worker is using separation from the group simply as a control device, he will not as a rule stay with the child, but simply send him off by himself for a short time until he can make a greater effort at self-control; discretion is needed in deciding when a child is ready for this kind of separation.

Deprivation of a pleasure or a privilege can be useful if the child feels that it is relevant to what he has done. We used an example above in which the child care worker said, "Do you think you are ready to go to the store this afternoon?" If the child thinks he is ready and goes on the trip, but cannot maintain control and has to be brought back early, the worker will probably draw the conclusion that he had misjudged the child's capacity to control himself and should not have given him the option of going to the store. He will not again take the youngster on an expedition on days when he has shown signs of similar upset, but he will not think of it as punishment. He will explain to the child that he feels he is not really capable of going to the store that day, substitute some pleasurable activity at the center, and do his best to help the child to think of the worker's decision as protection, not punishment. But at a time when he feels the child has control within his reach, as it were—and this is an intuitive decision on the part of the worker—he may say quite flatly, "No, I can't let you go to the store today because you grabbed the candy yesterday." He will still probably provide an activity at the center; the child will not have to mope around all afternoon with nothing to do. But having "the punishment fit the crime" makes it easier for the child to see it as the consequence of his misbehavior rather than as retribution or as an effort on the part of the worker to get even. He may still try to "put the adult in the punisher bag," as one worker puts it: "You're mean. You won't let me go. You don't like me." The worker cannot afford to be seduced into accepting this interpretation. A sense of humor can help at this point.

The recommendations in this chapter may seem complicated to any reader who is not already familiar with the atmosphere of a treatment center. To the experienced worker they only spell out in some little detail practices which he takes for granted and which combine to furnish an important part of the climate in which children can get better—a climate which offers tolerance and warmth, but also support and control.

CHAPTER 4

The Worker and Daily Care

At the end of the last chapter, we spoke of the climate that is created by the worker's attitude toward such matters as communication, response to feelings, and control of behavior. This chapter is devoted to the more routine aspects of child care. These comprise the worker's duties that affect the child's physical welfare, such as safety precautions or the provision for physical necessities including food, sleep, and cleanliness. Meeting these needs affects the children doubly: their bodily wants are satisfied, but also the way in which the worker insures safety, offers food, and manages the bedtime routine says something to them psychologically. The worker's attitude in these matters contributes to that important climate in which the children must grow just as much as does his attitude in more abstruse matters like verbal communication.

Safety

The child care worker must first of all care for the children's physical safety at all times. Safety is a concern in the care of any children but especially with children who sometimes seem unaware of ordinary dangers or who even try to hurt themselves. Disturbed children of any age may behave like babies in their disregard of hazards; they may climb to dangerous heights, put anything in their mouths, run into the street in front of trucks, or stick bobby pins in electric outlets. Some of them hit themselves repeatedly. Not all disturbed children do these things, and some of them are very timid and careful of their own safety; but even when the worker is thoroughly familiar with the child and his habits, nothing can be left to chance. The orientation procedures for workers in practically all treatment centers include some lessons in first aid, and if the population includes children who are subject to epileptic seizures, the workers are instructed in the measures to take to prevent a child from hurting himself during such a seizure.

Care for the children's safety includes preventing a child from deliberate self-injury, such as the head-banging or head-hitting that is sometimes seen but that can be overcome with adequate help. It also includes protecting a child from getting hurt by a more aggressive child. This does not mean interfering with all aggressive interaction between children. Aggression can at times mean progress, for the child who turns his aggression on himself needs to be helped to turn it outward. Ultimately the worker hopes that it may be channelled into constructive activity, into autonomy and achievement, but the first form it takes may very likely be an attack on another child. The worker has to protect the second child from injury, but to do it without forcing the first child to turn his aggression back on himself. The reader will recall that this subject was discussed in the section "Response to Feelings" in chapter 3.

Bathing, Dressing, Toileting

In residential treatment centers the workers are responsible for helping the youngsters to get up and dress in the morning and to get to bed at night. These duties include bathing them if they are small or are incapable of bathing themselves or perhaps helping them to bathe themselves. The workers may also have to help the children with toileting, to see that they get to the toilet at intervals if they are small or liable to toilet accidents, and to change them and clean up after them when they do have accidents. The worker should not think of this daily care as a chore to be got out of the way as fast as possible so that real "treatment" in the form of schooling or activities can begin. A good worker is able to use each event of daily care to help the child, and it is the quality of this care that makes one of the differences between milieu therapy and a custodial environment. Disturbed children come into treatment with substantial needs unmet, both the dependency need (the need for mothering) and the autonomy need (the need for establishing their own powers and abilities). Owing to their deep sense of worthlessness, they may have great difficulty both in accepting care and gratification and also in trying out their own powers. Careful planning for each child, with psychiatric direction, is desirable, but its success will depend on the acuteness of the workers' observations of the child's signals of his needs. He will indicate them, but he may do so in very tiny and obscure ways.

Some disturbed children have anxieties about bathing and toileting which they often cannot express but which may interfere with their performing these functions easily. Some are afraid, for instance, of the flushing of the toilet or of the draining of water from the tub, as though they, or some essential part of them, might go down the drain with the water. One nine-year-old boy used to leave the bathroom door open so if he fell in the workers would hear him yell and would come save him. Another child as he began to recover from his fears was able to say, "I thought the toilet was gonna bite me." Knowing that such fears are possible, the worker can be patient and not assume that the child is simply being stubborn. He can say something like, "I don't know just what it is you are afraid of, but you are safe; we'll take care of you and won't let anything hurt you." Such fears of the children should be reported in staff meeting and talked over with the psychiatrist or other supervisor. They are signs that the child has not yet developed basic trust in adults, and when the children are small and not very articulate, these fears are more likely to appear in the day-to-day situations involving bodily care than they are in the therapist's office. Only the older and more articulate children can tell the therapist, in words, what they are afraid of. For this reason, very young and very disturbed children are often not given individual therapy, but their treatment is dependent on a high quality of child care work with a high quality of supervision. Normal children when they are very small sometimes have fears such as have just been described, but they outgrow them because they gain more understanding and because they trust the adults who care for them. In the same way, but much more slowly, disturbed children can overcome their fears as the workers continue to reassure them and as they come to understand better the things around them.

Older disturbed children, who do not show the same signs of fear that the little ones do, often have developed rituals about bathing, toileting, bedtime, and getting up which have the function of warding off their fears. An example is the child in residential treatment who could not function in the morning unless he first went into the kitchen and had his morning juice; after that he could dress. Some rituals such as this one are not too far from the habits of ordinary children and indeed of adults and can be easily tolerated by the workers. More bizarre and time-consuming rituals, such as repeated handwashing, may require more patience on the part of the worker. The worker can acknowledge the importance of the ritual to the child and tell him that he hopes he will not always have to do it. Some children are afraid of being touched, and it is a sign of growing trust when they can ask for help from a worker. It should be added, too, that toilet training, like speech, will progress much faster if it is undertaken by the person who has the closest relationship to the child.

Occasionally a child whose toilet training has been rigid or punitive may need a period of regression before his development can go forward. Here it is not so much a question of anxiety as of a natural and normal stage of development which has not been fully lived through and to which the child returns to make up for lost time. He may need to soil himself a few times and perhaps even to play with the feces, as very small children sometimes do. This activity can be recognized by the workers as a necessity for this child at this particular time, and they can be permissive and understanding about it. The child will not regress permanently if he knows that the workers really have expectations for him to grow up, in his own way and his own time. If on the other hand the workers' basic feelings are that this child is not going to get better anyway, he is likely to regress and stay that way. It is important to remember that even normal children who are in the process of achieving toilet training are likely to relapse under stress—as the three-year-old does when a new baby comes into the family—and that they need affection and understanding, as well as expectations, to regain the lost ground.

Sometimes the child's anxieties are so great or his feelings of his own unworthiness are so strong that he resists all the worker's efforts to keep him clean and nicely dressed. He may refuse to be bathed, tear his clothing, smear his hair and clothes with dirt, and otherwise make himself as uncomfortable and unattractive as possible. The general rule for the worker in such cases is to handle the child as gently as possible but to insist on cleaning him up, reassuring him constantly that he, the worker, cares how he feels and wants him to enjoy being clean and comfortable. Cleanliness is for the child's sake, not for cleanliness's sake, and the child needs to understand, through the worker's actions as well as his words, that he is worth all this care. For special reasons the supervisor may advise letting a given child go around dirty when he wants to, but this is unlikely to be recommended often, for in most cases the child is likely to take it as a sign that he is not valued by the workers as highly as other children, even though he may have fought bitterly against the cleaning-up process.

A twelve-year-old boy in a children's residential unit so determinedly resisted his evening shower that eventually the workers, with the concurrence of the child's therapist, told him he need not take it unless he wished to. Most nights he did not wish to, but he confided in one of the workers that at home his mother did not make him take a bath, though she always made his younger brother take one, and that he regarded this as a sign that his mother loved his brother more than she did him. He had reproduced the home situation in the treatment center, not quite intentionally of course, but somehow hoping against hope that things would turn out differently there.

A compromise is often useful in such a situation. The worker can perhaps make a sort of contract with the child to take so many showers a week. It is not necessarily an either-or choice between letting the child go dirty or thrusting him bodily into the shower. The function of the treatment center is to demonstrate that people really care, that the world is not as he had previously experienced it.

Disturbed children who have never learned to wash or dress themselves or who have never been toilet trained can almost always gradually be taught these things if the workers devote enough time and patience to the effort. The decision when to urge self-care hinges on the worker's estimate of the child's needs for autonomy. Many children have a great longing to achieve competence in simple matters like dressing themselves but have never felt capable. It is a great deal easier to put a child's clothes on him than to stand by while he struggles to do the job, perhaps getting his pants on backwards and his shoes on the wrong feet. Or he seems not to hear at all the worker who is trying to get him to slip the T-shirt over his head but gazes far away into the distance, and perhaps only when he hears breakfast announced does he very quickly put it on and march into the dining room.

It is important not to expect too much too fast from any child and to raise the expectations by gradual stages, but always to have expectations. If a child seems to be teasing—and youngsters often do, especially as they are getting better—a little humor on the part of the worker may get a twinkle of laughter back from the child. A large part of the treatment of severely disturbed children consists of this kind of elementary education. What it does is help the child gain mastery of his world, something that normal children do as a matter of course but that disturbed children have been prevented from doing by their anxieties and by other factors in their lives. A child who, if he has had any concept of himself at all, has thought of himself as a baby who has had to have everything done for him or as a no-good character who could do nothing, now is able to think of himself as a person who can dress himself or as a person who can go to the bathroom by himself. His self-esteem is just that much higher, and this is a part of growth.

Times of bathing and dressing offer wonderful opportunities for workers with the younger children to play little games that mothers play with babies and toddlers but that these children have mostly not engaged in—games like This Little Piggy Went to Market, Shoe the Old Horse, Where Are Bobby's Ears, Where Are His Eyes? etc. Such games have the effect of making the child aware of his body and of assuring him that it is all there and that it is good, for disturbed children very often lack this awareness. Similarly, at any time of day a child who has developed some attachment to the workers can be helped to play games like Peekaboo and Hide and Seek, in order to play out his fear of being separated from the people he loves and to reassure himself that when people do disappear for a while they do in fact come back. As in the case of doing things for himself, the child only benefits when he enters into the game and enjoys it—a mechanical repetition is of no use at all. Resourceful child care workers will invent other kinds of games which will be of use to the children. It is good to bring them up for discussion in staff meetings so that the workers can fully understand what the games mean to the children. The workers soon get over any self-consciousness about discussing their activities and find that they can interact spontaneously with the children even though they report their interaction fully.

Food

Three meals a day, with snacks before bedtime and at any other time when they seem needed, is the rule in a treatment center. Food has emotional meaning for everyone. It is unconsciously equated with love; the baby's first experience of human love is the experience of being fed, and the giving of food is one

of the most important means of caring. Conversely, the withholding of food is an extremely drastic measure, since it is felt as a
withholding of love. Every decision about food in a treatment
center should be considered in the light of these facts.[1] It goes
without saying that the food offered the children should be palat-
able, the surroundings pleasant, and the atmosphere cheerful. It
is important first of all that the children should feel that the food
is lovingly given and that the workers are happy to see them
enjoy it. It is good if the children can sometimes ask for foods that
they particularly like and can sometimes plan the menu.

For many disturbed children the early feeding experience has
not been a satisfactory one, and they may have conflicts about
eating. Some children will eat only certain kinds of food, for
example, only baby food out of jars. Some have inhibitions about
chewing and will not take solids. Some will eat most kinds of food
but are totally unsocialized in their ways of eating—they may refuse to use silverware, make lightning grabs from other people's
plates, pour soup on the floor, and so forth. Older children are
sometimes worried about the cleanliness of the food or are afraid
that it is poisoned. Sometimes they will accept food only from
one special person, like the boy who before receiving treatment
would eat only dry cornflakes which had to be given to him by his
father who in turn could offer them only in the box so that they
would not be "dirty." Some children wolf anything and everything in great quantities, to the point of making themselves sick,
as though they could never get enough. There are individual reasons behind all these eating disturbances. As with the anxieties
about bodily care, they require discussion and understanding
among the staff, and patience, reassurance, and sometimes firmness on the part of the staff toward the children.

The messy eater who is otherwise fairly socialized is usually

1. The reader is referred to the excellent chapter on food in Morris Fritz
Mayer, *A Guide for Child Care Workers* (New York, 1958). No effort is
made here to cover all the relevant points but only to call attention to certain problems relating to food that arise in the care of severely disturbed
children.

more willing to socialize his eating habits when he knows that the workers like to have him enjoy the mealtime. It is sometimes helpful for such a child to have the worker say directly that he knows the child enjoys eating and that he approves of this enjoyment. With older children, setting up a "host" system is sometimes useful. The youngsters take turns being host. The host sits at the head of the table; gives seat assignments to the others; says when they will sit down, when they will start to eat, and when dessert will be served (but not *to whom* it will be served; everybody gets dessert). Taking turns at the host function brings in an element of competition which fairly competent children can tolerate well.

Totally unsocialized children, for whom the treatment goal is "habilitation" not rehabilitation, present a more complicated problem. For them enjoyment of eating—trying out and accepting a variety of foods, finding that it is fun to chew solid foods—is closely tied up with the development of trust in others and with the enjoyment of one's own growing powers. The workers' first task is to help the child develop this enjoyment; table manners, though important in the long run, are secondary to this. At the beginning of the treatment of an unsocialized child, workers should be prepared to tolerate almost anything in the way of bizarre eating habits, although from the first other children must be protected—for instance, a child who wants to snatch food from other people's plates can be made to understand that there are plenty of seconds for him but that he must keep his hands off other people's food. But, in general, mealtimes should be among the most permissive periods of the day precisely because it is so sensitive an emotional area for most of the children.

Each child should first be fully aware that the workers like to have him enjoy eating; only after that can they begin to help him socialize his eating habits. Nevertheless, this second step is important too; children should not be encouraged to go on month after month and year after year eating, for instance, spaghetti and mashed potatoes with their hands, although this method might have been tolerated when a given child was first in treatment. The food also should be plentiful, since any restriction in quantity is likely to be felt as a denial of love. This does not mean that a child should be allowed to gobble till he makes himself sick; such a child must be dealt with as a special case and a decision made as how best to help him help himself. Having the workers eat with the children, as is the practice in most treatment centers, is not only helpful in reassuring the children as to the goodness of the food but furnishes examples of table behavior which the children can gradually imitate. Above all, it creates an atmosphere of warmth and togetherness.

One day-care center for disturbed children introduced higher standards of table behavior at birthday parties than were permitted at ordinary lunch hours, with the reiteration, "This is a party, and so we will do so-and-so." At regular lunch hours, however, there were certain minimum standards, which were gradually raised as the children improved. Grabbing from one another's lunch boxes was discouraged from the beginning, but if a child wanted something that another child had, he could ask for it, offering something of his own in return. Since some of the children could not talk, some of the swaps were achieved nonverbally.

Sally, a nine-year-old nontalker, wanted one of Harry's corn curls, pointed to it, and held out her hand. He said, "You must give me something." She looked into her own lunch box, which was empty, and then got up and gave him a kiss. He ungallantly retorted, "A kiss isn't enough," but he gave her the corn curl anyway.

Food is a part of the ritual at birthday parties and holiday celebrations, and gradually the staff can help the children to build up the feeling that food is connected with pleasure and fun. When a kitchen is available to the children, a periodic cooking activity is useful to them and comes to be enjoyed more and more. Here they can take an active part—stirring, pouring, tasting, and then watching the mixture bubble on the stove or taking turns peeking into the oven while it bakes. Finally, they all can share in eating it. Few children can resist this kind of pleasure for long.

Sleep and Separation

In a private home after a bedtime ritual of some sort (maybe a bath, a story, a good-night kiss), the children are tucked into bed and expected not to be heard from till morning. In a treatment center where most of the children are fairly disturbed, at least one worker and maybe several are on duty and alert, for the children's uninterrupted night's sleep cannot be taken for granted. The anxieties that beset the children in the daytime may assert themselves even more strongly at night, and the lack of conventional behavior patterns shows itself sometimes in a disregard for the ordinary hours of waking and sleeping. Much can be done by the workers to prepare the way for a good night's rest for every child. The beds must be comfortable, the temperature of the rooms right, and the covers just enough for the season of the year. A bedtime ritual must be established that the children can count on and that is calming rather than exciting.

Children who have problems with control over their own behavior seem to fight sleep by being very boisterous at bedtime; it appears that they ward off sleep just because it represents a loss of control. At this time they particularly need to feel the strength of the adults, who firmly prevent their getting wild and insist on quieter behavior. The adult who says, "I'm just going to leave them alone" is not getting the children's message. If he lets the children grow wild at bedtime, he finds that they do not believe he can control them. His failure to intrude on their disruptive behavior may mean that the children can never go to sleep under his charge. The children may seem to prefer the more permissive handling, but they do not trust it.

There is of course a great advantage in having the same adult with the same group of children at bedtime, so that he and they can become accustomed to each other. A usual routine consists in baths for all, then a snack, and then tooth-brushing and bed—no roughhousing or chasing games for the last hour or so of the evening. Many children have their own private rituals at bedtime before they can settle down to sleep, as is indeed sometimes the case with normal children. A favorite toy can often help a child go to sleep, and the worker should not object if an older child wants to take to bed a hard toy, a truck, or gun, rather than the traditional cuddly animal. The worker's response to the youngster who wants to sleep with a toy pistol, for instance, is that he is glad that it helps him but that he, the worker, will be there too if the child needs him.

If several children share a room, assignments must be made with some attention to suitability. Since these are disturbed children, it cannot be expected that roommates will always live together comfortably, but as a minimum requirement children should not be put together who are likely to exploit one another. Workers must be prepared to have to minimize conflict—to do a great deal of negotiating and keeping of order. Children tend to keep one another awake in the best of circumstances, and a worker must often sit in the dormitory until all have dropped off to sleep.

Children must not be tucked in so firmly that it is difficult for them to get out of bed. A child must be able to get to the bathroom or to look for a worker if he feels afraid, and in any case a worker checks the rooms periodically to make sure that all is well. Just knowing that a worker is there and that he will look in from time to time may make it possible for a child to rest who might not do so otherwise. Sometimes a child cannot sleep because he is excited or upset over something that has happened during the day, and if he can tell the worker what is troubling him, he may be able to go to sleep.

Sometimes a disturbed child does not show any reluctance to go to sleep at night until he has begun to make a relationship with some adult among those around him, apparently because sleep is a separation from the person or persons that he has just learned to love. The night worker can reassure such a child that his favorite person will be there the next day or whenever it is that he is on duty again.

The separation problems that occur at bedtime should make us more alert to problems of separation that occur at other times of the day. Workers in most treatment centers make it a practice when they are going off duty to say good-by to the children and to tell them when they will be back, so that the children can count on them. They may also add, for the benefit of the children who seem more anxious about losing them, that so-and-so will be there and will take care of them while they themselves are gone. For some children, those for whom human relationships are new and therefore tenuous, reassurance is important when even brief separations occur. If the worker whom the children are most dependent on has to leave the group, for instance, to go to a meeting, he should tell the group that he has to be away for a short time and that another worker, so-and-so, will be taking care of them in his absence. Or such reassurance may be needed by one particular child more then by others:

Workers noticed that one seven-year-old became difficult to control whenever his regular worker left the room, even for a few minutes. He would sometimes try to prevent her leaving; he would stand in the door and kick or sit down and hang on to her ankle. His worker discovered that she had only to say to him, "I have to be gone for a minute, but Miss X. will take care of you while I am gone." He was then able to attach himself temporarily to the substitute worker, and his anxiety was lessened enough so that he maintained control of his behavior.

When a substitute worker takes charge of a group because of the illness of the regular worker, it may help a great deal if he says to the children, "I'll take care of you while Miss A. is away" and that Miss A. will be back "tomorrow" or "when she feels better," rather than just to report to them that Miss A. isn't here. These seem to be very small details, but they make a very great difference to the security of the children and to their improvement.

Care of Possessions and Use of Objects

One of the important tasks of the child care worker is either to care for the children's clothing and other possessions when the children are too young or too disturbed to care for them themselves, or to help in this task when the children, like most other children, are partly capable of looking after their own things but need some supervision. Workers are tempted sometimes to slight this obligation on the excuse that they are interested in the children themselves and not in "things." From the child's point of view, however, his bed, his dresser, his clothing, his books and toys all are extensions of himself, and to neglect these or to let them become lost or broken beyond the inevitable wear and tear is to diminish the child's sense of his own worth. The same is true of helping the child to define his "own" area, his "own" locker or drawer for his toys, his "own" clothes, his bed, his place at the table. He must be protected from indiscriminate use and destruction of his things by other children. These efforts on the part of the worker are techniques for helping the child define his individuality. This rule is even more important when the child does not seem to care at all about his own possessions; one means for the worker to help him gain a feeling for himself and his own worth is to care for his possessions and to keep assuring him that they *are* his.

Something of this attitude is important regarding the toys that belong to the whole group of children. It is terribly frustrating to a child who has just laboriously learned to put together a simple picture puzzle and who is enjoying the feeling of mastery to come into the playroom next day and find that one or two of the puzzle pieces have been swept up and thrown out with the trash. His achievement cannot be repeated for the puzzle is broken. What it means to him is that nobody really cares about his achievement and that it is hardly worth while to try again. Even the fact that a puzzle that one child has put together can later be taken apart so that another child may work it is a fact that may take some explanation and reassurance.

One little boy who had just finished a puzzle and had gone away briefly returned to find it scattered around the room. As he put it together again he repeated over and over, "Hide, hide, hide." After he finished he took his worker's hand and pointed to the top of a bookshelf, saying, "Johnny safe." In this poignant statement he indicated that something of his very self was invested in the completed puzzle and that to keep it safe was also to make him feel safer.

What the workers said and did about it is not part of the anecdote, but here was surely a challenge for them to demonstrate to him not only that for the time being they would certainly preserve his puzzle on the top of the bookshelf, but that in the long run they would always keep all the puzzle pieces intact so that he could repeat his achievement as often as he liked. Because children have such feelings, a separate drawer or locker for each child, where his things can be safe from the depredations of other children, is a real necessity; but such hiding places are of little use unless the workers use them properly, in full understanding of the importance of safeguarding the child's possessions and particularly the things he has made.

If a child is to be moved from one room to another, he should be on hand—to participate if possible but at any rate to witness— when his possessions are moved. Even if the change is one that he welcomes, it will require some adjustment; he may be restless and have sleep problems for a time after the move. If he is present during the move, he will feel less uprooted.

Older children who have a problem with behavioral controls are often destructive of their possessions. (This behavior seems to have some similarities to the withdrawn child's aimless manipulation of objects.) For the destructive child an opportunity to take objects apart and to put them together, with adult help, can be most useful. This task leads to a familiarity with the world of tools and to a growing sense of competency, less frustration, and less need for destructiveness.

Collecting objects that often seem to adults to be quite worthless is a favorite activity with normal children at a certain age. The more competent children among those in treatment often enjoy collecting "junk," and this activity is not to be offhandedly rejected by the workers, even though it may have to be limited at times if it gets out of hand. The size of the collection may be limited, if need be, but not the principle. Child care workers, like mothers, may sometimes be surprised at the worthless treasures that turn up among a child's possessions, but such hidden treasures often have meaning for the child.

The worker who is caring for severely disturbed, withdrawn children helps the child to structure his chaotic world by teaching him the use of objects. A skillful worker will first let the child explore an object in his own way, looking, handling, and perhaps even smelling and tasting, and then will gradually introduce him to the other possibilities of using it. Several centers which specialize in the treatment of severely disturbed children have found simple picture puzzles, form boards, and the like particularly useful in helping the children to master the concept of form and to gain some satisfaction in play. Since these children have skipped the usual playpen activity of very young normal children, of laboriously manipulating objects till they discover what fits into what and how toys work, they have to make up for missing this early stage of learning before they can go on to other forms of play and learning.

With or without special equipment, however, workers can make use of all the objects available in the center, clothing, furniture, eating utensils, and toys, to encourage children to try out, manipulate, and use. The meaning of objects dawns gradually. During one particularly successful camping trip a group of children who were quite disturbed were asked to fill and carry their own canteens full of water, although it was difficult to convey to them at first the reason for this requirement, and the canteens, in spite of all the verbal assurances of the staff, appeared from the children's point of view to be only so many meaningless objects. They tried to leave them behind or to pour out the water, but the staff insisted that they be both filled and carried in the expectation that the children's understanding, autonomy, and pride in achievement would gradually grow as a result of this expectation. The workers were rewarded for their efforts when a rather withdrawn child could finally say, "A canteen is for when you are thirsty."

If the worker can be mindful of the meaning to the children of these ordinary processes of daily living, the less glamorous parts of the residential or day-care program, many opportunities for encouraging growth can be discovered and used. For normal children these ordinary events are opportunities for learning and development, and we take this fact so much for granted that we give little thought to it. By taking a little thought, we can often help disturbed children to avail themselves of these opportunities.

CHAPTER 5

The Worker and Play

The Meaning of Games

Part IV of this volume is designed to help the worker in the task, which is often entirely his, of planning activities for the children during their free time. This chapter deals only with some of the values of free play and one or two other matters that may concern the worker in the small center.

As is pointed out in Part IV, children who are anxious and withdrawn seldom really seem to have fun. At most they seem to derive a certain satisfaction from the repetitious activities which they carry on, a satisfaction that appears to have more to do with security than with pleasure. Nor do the hyperactive or destructive children appear to get pleasure from their activities. They give the appearance of being constantly driven and rather frightened instead of satisfied by all their own activity. When children learn really to enjoy a trip, a game, or a party, or just to get pleasure from putting together a puzzle or mastering a simple task, they are getting better. As one experienced worker put it, the realization that "I'm having fun" can be just as exciting as the realization that "I can read."

Everyone, child or adult, needs some time to himself to pull himself together and think his own thoughts. In addition, for children who can make use of it, there should be time for free imaginative play or for games which they themselves initiate, since these are healthy, growth-producing activities. Naturally a higher proportion of the time will be allotted to planned activities in a day treatment center, where the children are present for only a few hours a day, than in a residential center, because it is assumed that the children will have ample time to devise their own activities when they go home. But even in a day center, periods of free choice of activity are important, their number and length being decided on the basis of a given child's need.

In a residential center, however, the periods when no activity is planned are as a rule too many and too long; there are long gaps of time between breakfast and school, between school and lunch, and so on through the day—far too much time for the children to use constructively unless they are able to take unusual initiative in organizing their own play. The way in which such gaps of time are used is a real test of the child care worker's art. Here is a time when the workers can make themselves fully available to the children for casual, relaxed interaction—conversation with the older and verbal children (even a game or a story if the waiting period is a long one), little informal games with the younger and less verbal ones, along with talk about what they have done earlier in the day or the evening before, what the plans are for the next activities, and the like.

The temptation for the workers is to let these in-between times be periods of empty waiting or to turn on a television, if available, and let the children watch whatever program is scheduled. These are easy "outs" for the workers and often antitherapeutic for the children. One of the reasons for bringing children to a treatment center is to secure for them a simplified, more easily understandable, and less frightening environment than the average child lives in. When they look at TV, they see things that are often confusing and often anxiety-producing—often violent. The directors of some treatment centers will not allow a television on the premises. In other centers, it is used only for the older and less disturbed children, and then only with a careful selection of programs. In any center that attempts to maintain a therapeutic atmosphere for the children, the TV should at the very least be in a locked room, not in the open living area where it can be turned on by anyone at will. When the children are taken in to see a program, the workers should be sure beforehand what the content of the program is likely to be and should be reasonably sure that it will be suitable for the individual children who are to see it. Even with the most careful choice, it is hard to predict the content of a television program, and even if the content seems benign, a child may view it as frightening.

Less disturbed children, though still disturbed enough to need day or residential treatment, can often play spontaneously by themselves or in groups. When we talk about children's play, we really mean several different things. One of these is the imaginative play that children engage in with toys or with each other, as when they play house, or milkman, or going to the doctor. Such play is in itself a sign of comparative health—the most deeply disturbed children are not capable of it—and it is often *autotherapeutic* to use Erik Erikson's term. This word means that children have a natural tendency to "play out" their anxieties and to help themselves cope with them in the process.

The role of the worker, when he sees such play going on in his group, is a delicate one. He will be aware in most cases that the play is healthy and constructive, so he will want it to go on. The inexperienced worker will be faced with two temptations. One is to turn his attention away since the children are taking care of themselves so constructively; the second is to intrude moralistically or to try to make the game a teaching vehicle, to make suggestions, to take a role himself, or at least to ask questions. No rule fits all circumstances, but if a good fantasy game is in progress, the temptation toward active intervention is usually to be resisted. The hardest role in such a situation is that of the "fly on the wall," the nonparticipant observer, but in most cases this is the role the worker should assume.[1] He should know what is going on, for this game may be very important because of its content, and he may want to discuss it in staff meeting; or it may lose its benign character—some child may be in danger of

1. There are certainly some exceptions to the general rule of nonintervention if the worker is trained in play therapy or for some other reason takes a more active role under the supervision of a psychiatrist. The *autotherapeutic* aspect of play is discussed by Erik H. Erikson in chapter 6 of his book *Childhood and Society* (New York, 1963).

getting hurt, physically or emotionally, and he may really need to intervene. If a question or two, quietly asked, will help the worker understand the content of the game better, perhaps he can venture that far, and certainly if he thinks somebody will be hurt he needs to interfere; but otherwise he should usually keep quiet, even if he does not entirely approve of the content of the game. For instance, the game may represent a good deal of conflict, and he may feel tempted to tell the children that people ought not to fight but to try to get along with each other. What the children are doing, however, is playing out the conflicts inside themselves that they cannot help having; if these conflicts can be worked out in play, they are that much less likely to make trouble in real life. Sometimes the children will ask the worker to take a role in a game, and then he may do so if he likes, but he should take care to keep to the role he is assigned and not put too much of his own fantasy into the game. Sometimes the game will show some serious misconception of fact on the children's part, and the worker can use his judgment about setting them straight.

In all cases it is good to bring a given child's play up for discussion in staff meetings or with child's therapist. It is an important index of what is going on within the child.

Lenny when he first came to school was obsessed with the story of Pinocchio and would call himself a puppet and ask to have strings put on his hands and feet. This was a perfect analogy to the way in which he was treated by his mother—as a puppet on a string. As time went on (he was now seven), he used his true dramatic ability to play-act for other children or just for himself. He gradually became less interested in Pinocchio, and more interested in the Wizard of Oz. He drew characters from this book and acted them out. One day he said, "At home I'm the Tin Man and at school I'm the Cowardly Lion." For quite a while he made lion costumes for himself and practiced roaring. He had made a paper wall for one of his plays, and finally one day he suddenly burst through the wall shouting, "I'm a boy! I'm a boy!"

Throughout the sequence of play, the workers had never intruded but had encouraged him by supplying properties as they were needed. The fact that he had an interested and sympathetic audience was certainly crucial in his creative use of play. At the denouement, when he declared himself a boy, the worker, who had never interpreted, did say warmly, "That's right! You are a boy!"

An aggressive hyperactive child in another center was given an opportunity for acting out his feelings in a legitimate way, the presence of the workers assuring him of control.

This ten-year-old, who was big for his age and had a severe behavior problem, would often try to hit people hard, blow after blow, especially toward the end of the day when he was about to go home. He was encouraged to play instead, and he devised a series of games involving destruction which he played with workers or with other children. He lived with grandparents who were extremely severe with him, and ultimately he was able to say that he was scared to go home, to which the worker responded, "I don't blame you for being scared to go."

When a child has to be removed from the group for a period because of aggressive behavior, an opportunity for him to play may be more useful to him than any effort on the worker's part to talk about what is troubling him. Though he may be able to assign some reason for his behavior—somebody perhaps did something to upset him—the deeper reason is probably beyond his knowledge.

A worker took a very aggressive ten-year-old, on one of his rougher days, alone into the yard with a basketball to get him away from the group. The youngster was too disorganized at that moment to play ball, but he was able after a time to start a game in which he was a tank and the worker was a cannon; the cannon had to hit the tank with the ball. Announcing that he was indestructible, the boy grunted, groaned, and clanked. Finally he said a tread had been knocked off, and he fell to the ground. The worker had to be the "tank retriever" and had to keep asking where he was broken. The game and the questions were repeated over and over, and the boy seemed to enjoy teasing the worker about his efforts to find out what was wrong. Finally the worker said, "This is sort of like being inside the center; you know and we know that you've got troubles, but we need you to tell us what's wrong." The youngster responded, "Yeah, I don't want to be in a place like this all my life."

A comment made in terms of the play itself, sensible but not moralistic, can often be useful.

A child who had good reason to be unsure of his mother's love invented a game in which he was a little puppy who ran away. The worker had to represent the mother dog and to call him back, saying, "I love you, I love you." The puppy would come back, but the child would say that it was all a trick, for the mother didn't really love the puppy.

A favorite worker was leaving her position, and was preparing the children for her going. This same child, playing that he was a puppy and she his mother, expressed his anger at her by saying, "I'm going to bite off your titties." Her very sensible response was, "If I were a mother dog and you were a puppy dog and you did that, I would really get angry."

An entirely different kind of play consists in games played according to rules, such as checkers or baseball. Here the worker often can and should take an active role to teach the children the game if necessary, to help them play according to whatever rules are agreed upon, and to help them with feelings centered around competition, success, failure, and other things that come up in the course of the game. Children who are just learning games are exposed for the first time to the rules of play. They may sometimes vary the rules at first because they do not yet understand them. But even after they know the rules, they may, like most other children of a certain age, want to vary them in their own favor in order to win. In a group game this naturally leads to conflict, and the worker will have to try to mediate. He may perhaps explain that the players can of course change the rules if they all can agree on the change. The rules as such are not important. What is important is that rules should apply equally to all players. It is far more important for the worker to bring about a compromise on which all the children can agree than to teach them the "real" rules of the game. The fact that they are able to come to an accommodation is the point; then the episode has been a real learning experience.

In a one-to-one game between a worker and a child, the same principle holds. There is nothing wrong with the worker's giving the child a handicap, if he plays much better than the child. And the rule book does not matter; they can make up any rules and play by them. But if the child insists on changing a rule in the middle of the game (because at that point it seems to his advantage to do so) the worker may say, "All right, we'll change the rule; we'll write it down, but then the same rule works for me." The child may complain or rebel, but when he really wins fairly, there is great triumph.

Although traditional games do not allow for the play of individual fantasy that is possible in free play, the worker should not make the mistake of thinking that traditional play is rational and innocuous. All play is potentially "loaded." Consider, for instance, the game of musical chairs, often played at parties, in which one child at a time is excluded from the group until only one is left. This game may be a very useful way for children to play out and cope with the feeling of being left out, and the feeling of coping with this anxiety may be one of the real, though unrecognized, sources of pleasure in this game, along with the competition, the suspense, the exercise of one's proficiency in darting for the empty seats, and whatever other elements may be in the game. But at a given time for a given child, for whom perhaps the feeling of being left out of the family group is too real and too close, this game may be altogether too much. One of the writers can recall observing a game of musical chairs where one little boy simply flew at the throat of his successful rival for the last chair.[2]

This chapter has attempted to give the beginning worker some

2. There is an instructive and entertaining analysis of the impulse and control elements in the game of Beatle in Fritz Redl, "The Impact of Game Ingredients on Children's Play Behavior," in *Fourth Josiah Macy Foundation Conference on Group Processes,* ed. Bertram Schaffner (New York, 1959).

awareness of the importance of play in children's development and specifically in that process of making up for retardation in development that disturbed children go through when they improve. Concrete suggestions for the worker in the planning of activities are offered in Part IV.

CHAPTER 6

The Worker and Group Relations

The Group of Children

The child care worker is almost always involved with a group of children rather than with an individual child. Even if at any given time he is working with a single child and is talking to him, he must be mindful of what is going on in the group and aware that everything he is saying to one child is heard by the others. An important habit for a worker to get into is never to have his back to the group unless absolutely necessary. Even if involved with a single child, he should position himself so that he has the whole group in view. Experienced child care workers even develop a sort of sixth sense about what is going on when they necessarily have their backs to the group, so that at the crucial moment they can turn around and attend to something that is going on across the room.[1]

Groups of disturbed children are typically staffed with at least two workers. Thus one worker can take a child out of the room for a short time if it seems to be necessary, because the child is too upset to stay with the group at the moment and needs a chance to calm down and perhaps to tell the worker what is bothering him, or perhaps because it is important to discuss with him out of the hearing of the group something that has just happened, or simply because the youngster needs someone to help him in

---

1. But as one of our helpful critics warns, don't assume you have this sixth sense unless you really have it.

the bathroom. Workers who are accustomed to cooperating with each other soon learn to read one another's nonverbal signals, so that much conversation is seldom necessary when they are actually with the children; discussions can be left till later when they are by themselves. When there are too many workers in the room for the number of children—as happens sometimes when there are students present—it is best not to allow each adult to occupy himself with a child, thus interfering with potential interaction among the children. Instead, some of the extra adults can withdraw to the sidelines and simply observe, allowing the children to interact among themselves, only taking a hand when asked to do so by the worker in charge. They should, however, always observe and listen. If a child detaches himself from the group and tries to involve one of the observers in one-to-one activity, the observer may remain friendly but should direct him back to the worker in charge or to the group.

The worker should form the habit of observing the group as a group at the same time that he observes each individual in it. It is often assumed that no real group formation is possible with children who are so severely disturbed that very little communication goes on among them, but anyone who takes the trouble to watch such a group long enough will realize that there is indeed a group sense, that individuals do play varying roles within the group, and that the children seem very much aware of the group as a group. The child who shows anxiety when any other child is missing is one example of this awareness. Observers have sometimes noted a sort of division of space among severely disturbed, isolated children. The seeming prearrangement by which two children "exchange corners" is one such example. One worker reports that a room was tacitly divided into five "territories" by five nonverbal children, each of them occupied with his own compulsive play and seemingly unaware of the others but never encroaching on their space. Extended observation will show that there is a certain division of roles even among the most withdrawn children, with one child often expressing anxiety for the whole group in times of stress.

One of the writers has seen a nonverbal child, seemingly the most withdrawn of his group of five, repeatedly instigate behavior that the worker was trying to discourage. The worker had got all five children settled in their dormitory for the night. This child, who had a repertoire of sounds, would call out some incomprehensible syllables, and the four others would begin to bounce on their beds. The worker would make the rounds and tuck them all in, and all would be quiet for a few minutes. Then would come the same call from the same child, and the bouncing would start all over. The one who was doing the calling did not bounce but limited himself to giving the signal to the others.

This is the kind of situation that calls forth from an experienced worker what someone has termed the *hooray-damn response*. On the one hand, the worker was delighted to see these withdrawn children interacting as a group and to see the most withdrawn functioning as the leader. On the other hand, it was long after their bedtime, and it was most inconvenient to have them bouncing around like that. Besides, they would all be tired and cross the next morning.

In this example the children had formed their own group and had set themselves playfully against the intentions of the worker. Almost certainly, however, the children were able to interact in this way only because of her presence. The worker needs to form the habit of thinking of himself in a sense as a member of the group and in most circumstances as its leader. "If you're there," one worker says, "you're part of the interaction." As leader, the worker accepts all members of the group for what they are; he does not play one against the other but helps all the children to interact with himself and with one another. When a decision is to be made in which the children can participate, he encourages all to share in making it, not just the few who are vocal. Perhaps he says to them, "Where do we want to go today?" A good many of the children are screaming their suggestions at once. The worker says, "I hear 'zoo'; I hear 'park'; I hear 'stay here.' How are we going to work it out?" Someone suggests that they take a vote. All those who want to go to the park are asked to raise their hands. Some of the nonverbal children raise their hands to indicate their preference for the park. Eddie, nonverbal, has with-drawn from the group and is lying under a bench. What does Eddie want to do? Thomas, who talks very well, gets down on his hands and knees beside Eddie. "I think he votes yes," he reports. It does not matter whether Thomas's opinion is correct or colored by his own preferences; at least everyone knows that Eddie's wishes are important too. One worker with a group of such children was successful in getting one or two, who had almost no speech, to pronounce the single word that showed their preference about the evening's activity. Being included as effective group members elicited what little speech they had.

As the children begin to feel more and more that they are parts of a healthy, functioning group, they take on the adults' attitude that every member is important and worthy of respect. Thomas, in the example above, when he tried to consult the opinion of the deeply regressed Eddie, showed this attitude. In a different kind of group a regressed child of such unsocialized behavior might have been laughed at and picked on. As time goes on, if the group attitude is good, children begin to help one another. If one child sees that another needs help beyond what he himself can give, he may call an adult's attention to the matter. In one group a child who was just learning to speak, noticing that one of the other children was becoming very upset, summoned the worker with the anxious words, "Louis [the other child]—quiet room!"

A similar task confronts the worker when he has a group with a number of disruptive children in it and one child assumes the role of group bully. Although the worker's presence prevents overt abuse of other children by this one child, the dominance structure of the group is very clear. Such a dominating child typically develops a friend who plays the role of "bully's assistant." Typically also one child is selected as "victim." When group decisions are to be made, even in the presence of the worker and with his participation, the bully and his assistant may declare their wishes loudly so that the other children may be too intimidated to speak up and may even insist that they have no other wishes than those which have been expressed for them by the bully. (As a rather naïve worker once put it, "Of course they like him best because he is the strongest.")

The worker naturally wants to make the group structure less rigid. He may try to bring about some exchange of roles when group decisions are made, such as having children take turns in suggesting or planning activities. He will also look for games in which an exchange of roles is mandatory, for instance, in which the person who pursues at one time becomes the person who is pursued at another (as in Prisoner's Base) or in which a leadership position rotates among the children and all have to do what the leader directs (as in Simon Says or Mother, May I?)

One worker found it very useful to talk separately to the two children who were the bully and the victim about each other. Not only did Ted at times have to be punished for his behavior toward Jim, but the worker had also to sympathize with him because Jim seemed to tempt him into bullying behavior. He had to realize, in effect, that he did not need to let Jim make him be such a bad boy. On the other hand, Jim, who was dominated and tormented by Ted, had to realize that this could only happen because he allowed it. It took him a long time to recognize his anger against Ted, but eventually he did so. Each became more independent and the bullying tapered off. During this process the worker was careful to arrange some times when the two children did not play together but interacted with other youngsters, thus getting the opportunity to try out new roles within the group.

As with the withdrawn children described earlier, a group made up largely of acting-out youngsters may slowly develop attitudes of mutual helpfulness. In one group which included varying kinds of disturbances, a child with bullying tendencies, even before he had overcome the need to torment a victim, showed great compassion toward an extremely withdrawn child and made great efforts to help him. Later he was able to extend this attitude to other members of the group, and because he occupied a position of leadership, he was imitated by the others.

Whereas in a group of verbal children, who will usually interact freely, the worker will be chiefly concerned with the kind of interaction that occurs, in a more withdrawn group he may have to be alert to notice any signs of interaction and be careful not to interfere with it. He will learn the art of pulling back to permit the interaction that will occur more and more as the children begin to function as a group. Sometimes when the children attempt to interact with the worker, he can redirect them into interaction with other children. One worker reports that for the sake of the rest of the group she deliberately does some limit-setting in the presence of the whole group—that is, a child whose behavior is unacceptable is not always taken out of the room before she talks to him. When a child runs away, kicks a worker, or masturbates in front of the group, the other children wonder, "What is the worker going to do?" and it may be important that she deal with the child in front of the others so that their need to know is satisfied. (There are other times, of course, when it is necessary to take the child off by himself.) The episode recounted in chapter 3 in which a quite competent, almost-well child who had deliberately broken a window was sent home for the rest of the day spoke more loudly to the rest of the group than a whole dissertation.

It requires a sharp eye at times to distinguish which child is really instigating trouble; it may not be the one who is really doing the misbehaving. Careful observation is often required to be sure what the group structure actually is at a given time, who is assuming leadership, and who is following.

In one group the most withdrawn child assumed a sort of leadership at rest time, for he was best able to rest quietly. When on one occasion he apparently tried to exploit this leadership position by getting up and walking conspicuously around among the children, the worker was able to point out humorously to the group what the boy was trying to do, "supporting" him in a sense and not insisting that he lie down, but also pointing out that none of the others followed his example. She felt that on this occasion the other children saw him in a new light for the first time. They also accepted her different handling of this child; he was permitted to walk around because he needed to, whereas all the others had to rest.

This is another of the benefits of a good group climate. Children can accept the fact that different members have different requirements ("He needs this right now") and that all need not have identical handling.

The Workers' Feelings and the Group of Workers

The atmosphere in the children's group is directly influenced by the atmosphere in the group of workers. The way in which the worker handles his feelings is important to the children. Child care workers have to be child-loving and child-respecting people in order to enter the profession at all, but any children can try the patience of adults at times, and disturbed children, with their extreme negativism and their sometimes uncivilized ways, can often make an adult angry. With experience the worker does build up a kind of tolerance; he gets angry less easily. But there are still times, particularly when the worker finds his physical reserves pushed to the limit or when he becomes unbearably anxious about what is happening, when he may find his self-control taxed. He may try to conceal his feelings from the children, but children are past masters at seeing through a façade, and they are likely to push an adult further and further until he reveals something of his real emotion. When the adult feels that his patience is wearing out, it is better for him to let the children know something of what he honestly feels. "Yelling" at a child is not invariably a mistake, but he must not "let go" to the point of hurting the child verbally or physically. It is at times like this when adults are tempted to yank too hard or hold too tightly. If he can, the worker may try to avoid getting physically involved with a child when he is this angry. He may be able to ask another worker to take over for him temporarily so that he may go somewhere and cool off. But sometimes there is no other worker at hand, and he is compelled to tangle with the child to prevent something worse from happening, and in this case he simply does the best he can. If his performance is not perfect, he need not feel too guilty. Afterward, when he and the child both have cooled off, they can talk over what happened.

The beginning worker immediately notices that some of the children in the group are much easier for him to like and sympathize with than others; he may notice that there is one child who particularly exasperates him. These feelings on the part of the worker are important. He often feels that he can understand, and thus reach and influence, a child for whom he has special sympathy. But there is a danger too. If a worker is tempted by his feelings into showing favoritism, not only is it hard for the child whom he favors, but he loses his power to influence the rest of the group. Often too there is some one child in the group whom it is particularly hard to like because he seems bent, full time, on showing his ugliest and most exasperating behavior. The worker has to remember that this is not what the child *is*, this is the way in which he is behaving; somewhere behind the ugly brattish actions is the real child who both wants and needs a positive relation with adults. If a worker responds to a given child with an unusual amount of annoyance, it is often because the child's behavior stirs up some less mature part of himself—and everyone has such parts. When this happens, the worker cannot be very useful to the child unless he comes to understand what has been stirred in himself. Supervision may sometimes help workers to come more rapidly to an awareness of what it is that is stirring.

It is helpful to realize that the children's behavior, positive or negative, is often not really directed at the worker as a person. The children use the worker for their own needs, and whether he is treated lovingly or angrily, he must learn to accept it and not take it too personally.

One little girl in a treatment center selected two of the women staff members as the targets respectively of her angry and loving feelings. One of them, her own worker, she continually attacked, often physically, trying to bite and kick her; to the other, a worker in another but accessible group, she showed her sweetest and most feminine side. True, there was some rational basis for the child's choice. Her own worker was necessarily very much aware of the little girl's need for control, and being in charge of the group, she had the task of controlling her. The other worker responded somewhat more freely to the child's need for indulgence. It was probably important to the little girl at that time to have these different needs filled by different people, so that she could sort out the ambivalent feelings that she had for her own mother. Since both staff members were experienced, they maintained the integrity of their own relationship, and each accepted her role as the child had defined it. After many months of "working through," the child was able to bring the negative and positive feelings together and express both appropriately to her own worker, the one who had received the negative treatment but who was the one, like her mother, the child most wanted to be close to. The child and the other worker remained good friends, but finally the child could show anger toward this worker, too, as well as affection. Both relationships were realistic and genuine. The ambivalence was manageable, as it is with normal children.

This subtle interplay of feelings between children and staff, particularly the feelings of staff members themselves, can cause much trouble and confusion unless it is carefully evaluated. It furnishes much of the subject matter for supervisory conferences and staff meetings. Staff members need not be ashamed of having feelings about the children, even very strong ones; if they did not have feelings, they could not help the children. The feelings that go back and forth between the children and the adults help to provide the ladder by which the children can climb out of their disturbances.

Feelings among staff members are important and affect the structure of the worker group and the quality of the work with the children. Every human being has both positive and negative qualities; and when people work together as closely as they must in a treatment setting, their whole personalities become involved, not just their polite superficial side. As one professional has said, "In this work, everyone's slip is showing from time to time." Thus annoyances arise, as well as honest differences of opinion. These things must be dealt with in staff meetings or in one-to-one discussions, or else they may adversely affect the work with the children. Children are quick to pick up a feeling of strain or of unworked-out controversy among adults.

Some children are proficient at playing one adult against another, if the adults are not alert for this. They may, for instance, ask permission from one adult for something they want and then if it is denied apply to another adult without revealing that they have already asked the other. Child care workers, like good parents, learn to check with each other first, to make sure they are giving reasonably consistent answers. The child sometimes does not even really want the thing he has asked for but gets his satisfaction from upsetting somebody. The workers can recognize his manipulation without offense and without "putting the child down"—without being his victim and without victimizing him. Here again a bit of humor often helps.

Basic lack of respect between workers can be even more damaging than lack of consistency. Workers and all team members owe it to the children to study the structure and dynamics of their own group and to work hard to establish an atmosphere of trust among themselves. With enough good will it can usually be done.

Chapter 1 emphasized the fact that if an atmosphere of trust is to be maintained among the workers, continual communication is necessary. In the following chapter it was pointed out that for the very practical reason of passing around the information needed for the best care of the children, communication is also necessary. The chapter described the number and kinds of meetings which are planned in many centers for the passing back and forth of this information. Here both these points should be reemphasized. If workers are to come to an agreement about differences of opinion, there must be a time and place for them to talk together. Likewise if a child has been upset on a visit home and the parent counselor has heard about it, the workers must know it at once, so that they can help the child with his feelings. If, on the other hand, the child tells the workers of some event on his visit home that has been upsetting, they must get the information to the child's therapist and the parent counselor as soon as possible, so that a common policy can be decided on and carried out. Similarly, things may have happened in the residential setting which may be important for the counselor to communicate to the parents.

One of the most frequent defects in child care settings is the simple failure of all adults at all levels to pass such important information back and forth. This usually comes about because workers, and too often their supervisors also, are so overwhelmed by the pressures of managing the children that they consider communication a luxury. Meetings may be too infrequent and too highly structured for the exchange of detailed information about the children's daily lives. But communication is a necessity, not a luxury, if the children are to be effectively managed; and only this detailed exchange of information will enable each worker to know enough about each child to do his best for him. The continual passing back and forth of the tiny bits and pieces of facts about the children's daily lives is one of the requirements of child care work; otherwise many therapeutic opportunities are missed, and untherapeutic accidents occur for sheer lack of information.

PART III

Child Care Work
in the Large Institution

by Karen Dahlberg VanderVen, with Contributions
by George M. Cohen and Genevieve W. Foster

CHAPTER 7

The Worker and the Institutional Program

The Children

What types of children usually find their way into large institutions? Often institutionalized children are among the most severely disturbed, for whom outpatient treatment or day treatment has not succeeded or would not reach the depth of their disturbances. The worker would be likely to find some highly withdrawn children, often with little or no speech, along with other psychotic children, severely disturbed though verbal, whose behavior may be extremely bizarre and disorganized.

The so-called "acting-out" children may be found too. These children may be very verbal, but are more accustomed to expressing their feelings about themselves and the world through angry behavior such as swearing, destroying property, fighting, precocious sexual behavior, and stealing. Such children have often come from multiproblem families whose difficulties include poverty, disorganization, marital disruption, and all the conditions which contribute to family breakdown and poor emotional climate for children to develop in. It should be emphasized, however, that by no means do all the children come from such families. The families of many are loving and committed, and the factors that have brought them to the institution do not include neglect. Other more obscure and sometimes unknown factors account for their deviances.

Finally, there is the child with multiple disabilities. This child may have a physical problem and/or be mentally retarded in addition to being emotionally disturbed, with all conditions contributing to the events leading to his institutionalization.

Many of the children who come to residential care have had an irregular and inadequate program of physical care. Most of those for whom this is true are the children from multiproblem homes, though others have resisted the best efforts of their families to establish good regimes for them. Their sleeping hours have perhaps been chaotic, their diet poor in nourishment, their medical and dental supervision greatly lacking. Some may not have had serviceable or clean clothing; some may have roamed the streets at all hours. These are children for whom the order and regularity of an institution—three nourishing meals a day, one's own bed, daily care, protection from the mistreatment of older children—constitute therapeutic factors in themselves.

The institution, then, can offer a wholesome pattern of daily living. In the institution the general framework—meals, sleep, toileting, etc.—is helpful for many children in building them up physically and increasing their resources for learning and for working on their emotional problems. With their medical-nursing administrative organization, many institutions such as state hospitals can offer fine medical care and supervision to their children right on the grounds.

Again, many children who have come into institutions have had extremely chaotic relationships with people within the framework of their highly disorganized families. They may have experienced violence, neglect, seductive sexual activity, unusual responsibilities, and generally inconsistent or inappropriate handling. Although sometimes the handling of children in institutions may lack (from the child care point of view) warmth, consistency, and understanding, it may be more caring and consistent than that experienced previously by children with this kind of background. The institution provides a structure for relationships which the child may never have had before. There are usually in institutions many staff members who, whether or not they are highly trained, care deeply about the children in their charge, who are warm, and who offer stable figures for identification.

Before being placed in the institution, severely psychotic or acting-out children have usually not had recent schooling, because of their unacceptable behavior and poor functioning in the public-school classroom. Although there might not be as much educational programming as one would like within institutions, the school program is still one of its most effective offerings. Many more institutionalized children have more opportunity for some schooling than they would have had in the community, and the program is much more tailored to their educational and behavioral difficulties. Thus a real advantage of many institutional programs for children is the intramural school.

Before institutionalization many severely disturbed children have had little or no opportunity for group play and interaction with other children. Out of school they were different from other children in the neighborhood and thus excluded from their groups, and so they have had little social contact with others of their age, or else they were bullied and scapegoated. If their placement in an institution is appropriate, there will be other children similar to them in age and functioning, so that perhaps for the first time in their lives they will have real peer companionship. More and more those in charge of institutional admissions are attempting to ensure that no child is alone in the sense that he does not have other children like himself to relate to and thus would suffer a big gap in his developmental environment.

To sum up, institutional programs can offer children, particularly those whose previous lives have been deprived and chaotic, many experiences that are restitution for some of these lacks. The activity program, the school program, and the everyday aspects of unit living, all contribute to the benefits. The staff members who help a child learn to brush his teeth, who help him build a house with a construction toy, who take him roller-skating or on a trip to a dairy, who let him help prepare the evening snack, who help him learn to play with other children, all are helping to make up for important experiences that each one has missed.

The Child Care Function in the Larger Setting

The child care worker who has been trained in smaller settings but who begins work in a large institution will soon notice differ-

ences between the two. In the small setting the child care worker
may have found himself responsible for perhaps five or six children who were somewhat alike in general disturbance and functioning. An insitutional worker may occasionally have so few, but
much of the time he may have fifteen to twenty-five children
under his aegis. At times he may work by himself, but usually he
is serving on a tour of duty in company with one or, if he is lucky,
two other child care workers, depending on the size and nature
of the group. The children may be similar in age and disturbance,
but more likely they will be different—younger, older; verbal,
nonverbal; active, passive—all living together on the same unit.

The child care worker who has served in a residential unit will
be familiar with the shift system; but one whose experience has
been in day treatment will see that a residential institution, being
responsible for caring for the children twenty-four hours a day,
seven days a week, must have shifts of workers to relieve each
other. An exception is the residential center utilizing live-in cottage parents. Most institutions, like the smaller centers described
in chapter 2, run on shifts from 7:00 A.M. to 3:00 P.M., 3:00 to
11:00 P.M., and 11:00 P.M. to 7:00 A.M. This set-up, however, provides some interesting problems; for example, it is usually impossible for all the child care staff to meet together. Other aspects
will be discussed in the section on communication in chapter 11.

Whereas the worker coming from a small center once worked
closely and informally with a small group of people whose functions were more or less like his own, in the institution he may
find himself a member of a department with specific duties. For
example, in the small center the worker may have shared in planning and carrying out the entire daily program, including crafts,
work activities, and daily routines. In the institution he may find
that his formal responsibilities are for physical and "home" care,
while such units as the occupational therapy, recreational therapy,
and activities departments take some of the children off the living
area for certain periods of time for games, crafts, trips, etc. If, on
the other hand, the child care worker is employed not on the
living unit but as a member of one of these departments, he will

not be responsible for such aspects of care as dressing or feeding the children. Usually a trained child care worker is a member of the child care staff—those individuals who take care of the children on the living units, the area where the children sleep, eat, dress, rest, and spend many hours when they are not at school, out on visits, or engaged in other activities.

The special approach of child care, with its understanding of the developmental needs of children, is highly appropriate in the living unit. It is needed, however, in any department that deals with children. There is a certain overlapping of functions between the various departments of an institution. Child care workers on the living unit find that to be most effective they need to develop activity programs right on the unit, either for the children who are not picked up by other departments or for the children who spend time with other departments but still have many free hours in their living areas. Conversely, activity workers inevitably are involved in some physical care of the children, as they get dressed for swimming, eat on picnics, scrape their knees during a baseball game, etc. And in conducting the activities themselves, the activity workers need to understand the developmental needs of the children as well as something of their psychopathology. Some institutions have met this problem by providing a child care worker with special training in activities who is geographically based in the living unit rather than in some special part of the institution, serves as resource person to the rest of the staff, and assumes leadership in the matter of recreation, crafts, and organized games.

The concerns of the institutional child care worker involve both overall and specific duties relevant to creating a therapeutic living situation for the children. Life for the children, because it is lived in groups within an unnatural physical and child-rearing environment, may become destructive to their growth unless the staff members, including the child care workers, make concentrated efforts to meet the special needs of children within the framework of the institutional program.

Treating Children as Individuals

One feature of institutional living is the frequent lack of privacy and the resultant lack of dignity for the residents. This problem is exemplified by locked bedrooms, communal bathrooms and bathing procedures, lack of individual storage space, lack of individual property, etc. Although some aspects cannot be changed—and some, in the interests of safety, should not be—if the worker is aware of them, he can often help to institute some practices which restore individual dignity to the children. Boys can make boxes for their belongings in woodshop. The entire unit of children can participate in a project of stenciling designs on curtains which might serve as window or toilet-stall curtains or as room dividers.

Why is maintenance of dignity so important? Studies in psychiatric treatment indicate that mental patients receive much feedback from their status—from the way in which they are viewed by the staff, from what the staff say and do, and from their physical surroundings—and that this feedback contributes to their response to treatment and their ability to get well. If they are assured of their worth, they respond more favorably. Children also achieve and develop their identity in part through what the physical setting "tells" them about what they are like and what is expected of them.

In group living one needs to be aware that each child is a unique individual and should be so considered in planning programs, methods of handling, and relationships. A large and varied group may challenge the ingenuity of the child care worker, but he *can* help see that each child gets individual consideration. One child may often need the opportunity to be alone so that he can gather his resources or even face the anxiety he usually avoids by making himself the hub of group activity. Another child in the same group may need continual encouragement to come out of his isolation and be with others. For one child speaking firmly may help him regain his self-control. For another this may serve only to upset him further. The child care worker may group similar children together at times so that the general method of handling meets the needs of all members; at other times he may group dissimilar children so that they can stimulate one another.

In a large group it is easy sometimes for a worker to find himself responding more to some children than others, to find himself paying more attention to the verbal active children who actually demand it than to the quiet ones. Or he may find himself tending to be highly interested in just one child to the exclusion of the rest. It goes without saying that anyone who works with children naturally finds himself more attracted to some children than others, and if the worker is aware of this problem, he can prevent it from altering his effectiveness. (This was touched on in the discussion of the workers' feelings in chapter 6.) Despite the worker's preferences, it is important that each child receive equal consideration from the staff although one may not be as appealing, demanding, or responsive as another. The need for attention of the withdrawn children, especially, may be masked by their passivity. The worker who really wants to help all the children will try to devise ways of giving his interest to these children who try so hard to fend off attention but really need it to get better. There can be few things more gratifying in work with children than observing a new accomplishment from one of these withdrawn children and realizing that it might not have occurred without the effort of the worker.

It is often the case in institutions that there are so many ready-made rules and procedures that there is little apparent flexibility and little opportunity for the children to make choices and to weigh alternatives. In hospitalized adults one often hears of "institutionalization"; they have become so accustomed to following a rigid regime that they are afraid to leave the hospital where they have not had to assume their own direction of their daily lives. This is not to say by any means that children should assume entire responsibility for the way things are run or that they should define how their unit is set up. They do not, of course, have the resources for this. But a surprising amount of choice can be offered without disrupting hospital policy or rules. Instead of an adult's selecting and laying clothes out ahead of time, he could ask, "Would you rather wear your red or your blue shirt today?" or, for boys, "Would you rather have your hair longer or a crew cut?" instead of insisting on the standard cut for all.

Carrying out this idea of decision-making for the children is a subtle thing sometimes; with withdrawn children especially larger decisions about participation, for example, must be made for them. Of their own choice they would remain isolated, but this decision would not help them learn to deal with reality or to get along with people. They would not be asked whether they want to help clean up the playroom—their participation would be required—but they might be encouraged to choose whether they will pick up papers or wipe the table.

In group living, as we have said above, children need to be placed so that they have the opportunity to associate with some other children similar in age and development. One sometimes hears of adolescents living on adult units because there is no other place for them, of a lone withdrawn child on a unit of acting-out children, etc. A judicious mixing of children can be therapeutic—it is analogous to family-style living—but in general each child should have an opportunity to live with one or more children similar to himself in age and functioning.

Programming for Daily Living

The Need for Program

Even more than normal children, institutionalized children need growth-producing activity and program appropriate to their age, emotional status, ability, and treatment needs. This is in many ways an untapped area in the field of child care, since it seems that on many units even those trained child care workers who understand group dynamics and individual feelings may not know how to organize constructive individual group play and activity.

A full activity diet for children is important not only because it "keeps the child busy and out of mischief"—although for industrious workers these results also can be useful—but because it is a key element in the growth and development of children, who achieve through play experience their mastery of the physical and social world. In institutions where there is little program, the children spend their time in angry, dissipating boredom, and the staff members by necessity expend much punitive effort to control them. In other institutions there might be a good program for the verbal, active children while the passive ones languish unoccupied. The staff may rationalize about these children: "But they don't want to do anything else." This may well be true, but they need activity program just as the others do, and they need special handling and support in order to participate in and profit from it. Frequently a large responsibility for programming for withdrawn children is devolved to the child care worker, and a succeeding section of this chapter will discuss this task in more detail.

We have been speaking of program in the specific sense of play and recreation, but program in the larger sense is also important. One of the greatest weaknesses in institutional life, one which accounts for much destruction, aggression, hyperactivity, unhappiness, and lack of development in the children, can be the lack of special planning required for a good living situation for children. What this means in general is that there is little or no pattern of organization in living for some children, especially the more withdrawn ones. The days may be spent in a gray area of bland or nonexistent stimulation, aside from time spent going to meals, getting ready for bed, etc., with the bland stimulation consisting, perhaps, of adult hustle and bustle, some noise from other children, and the drone of the TV in the background.

The need for program is related to the previously mentioned need of institutionalized children to develop and maintain an individual identity, a sense of mastery, and a sense of worth as a person. In a large setting where there is not really the opportunity for great amounts of time to be spent in individual work with children, the program often provides the means by which this need is met. Through the meaningful organization of the day and through their participation in the activities offered, the children have a chance to develop and display new skills, and these contribute to their sense of personal worth.

Use of Time-Space Structure

How then can the child care worker develop a more growth-producing and indeed more pleasant living situation for the children in his care? From the practical point of view, there are a number of basic principles he can consider. A key concept is that of "structure." Often grim faces are made when this word is heard, for it may conjure up images of regimented activities in which children must do precisely as adults say in a rapid succession of highly planned and inflexible programs. It is undoubtedly true that it is possible to overstructure children's lives and activities, but nevertheless the concept of structure has many therapeutic possibilities when applied to institutional living if the structure is created around the needs of children.

In some recent literature concerned with therapeutic milieus, the "time-space" concept is described as a meaningful way of imposing structure on the ongoing life in treatment centers.[1] This means that routines, activities, and other aspects of unit life are designed and developed so that the passage of time is broken up into discrete units appropriate to the needs and tolerance of the children, and large spaces are broken up into smaller, functionally defined areas.

To impose a time structure, there can be scheduled periods for many activities—outdoor time, snack time, rest time, TV time, cleanup time, activity time, etc. One conceptual area in which almost all disturbed children, particularly the withdrawn, are sorely deficient is in the ability to experience time accurately. To orient themselves to the reality of the current moment, there are many aspects of time which they must understand. If they themselves cannot do this, an environment that will help them do it must be created by dividing time up into discrete units. This

1. John Cumming and Elaine Cumming, *Ego and Milieu: Theory and Practice of Environmental Therapy* (New York, 1962), pp. 89–105.

makes the environment more predictable, hence more anxiety reducing. The children can operate more effectively in it and derive greater benefit from it. Also, to help the children orient themselves in time, such mechanical props can be utilized as calendars on which children can mark off the days as they go by and posted schedules of activities and appointments for each child. It is a good plan to sit down with the children after breakfast and talk with them about what they are going to do that day, even though they might have been told previously.

Concomitant with the structuring of time is the structuring of space. All of us are aware of the fact that we unconsciously behave differently depending on the immediate physical setting, that a small carpeted room, for instance, calls forth a different type of response from that evoked by a large bare gymnasium. The same principle applies to the behavior of disturbed children. Large undefined spaces invite feelings of confusion and a sense of spatial disorganization which provoke anxiety as the youngsters seek a stable orientation. If this acclimation is provided by the environment, the children are able to function more appropriately and effectively.

It has been mentioned already that in some institutions the arrangement of physical space is less than ideal. There may be long dark corridors which invite aimless pacing, sparsely furnished group or dayrooms which invite wall sitting, poorly located bathrooms, difficult access to the out-of-doors, etc. Poor basic arrangements, of course, make things difficult for both staff and children, but the difficulties can be circumvented to some extent by clever management. One fairly large area can be left free for active games. All other spaces can be broken down by rearranging furniture; putting up partitions and hangings; setting up "corners" appropriate for different activities; and, most specifically, establishing designated functions for different areas and showing by signs, furnishings, and materials (as well as by talking with the children) what they are to be used for. Extra rooms can be turned, for example, into game rooms for the more verbal children, who need a place where they can play peacefully, work on hobbies, talk quietly with one another, and be alone. The withdrawn children need, perhaps, a playroom where there is large-muscle-developing equipment, strong safe play materials such as balls, and a cupboard accessible to staff with basic arts and crafts materials.

In subdividing the space, it is important to avoid flimsy plywood or composition partitions; these can be too easily broken down by the children, with resulting feelings of guilt. If these are all that are available, it is better simply to rely on an arrangement of furniture or of sturdy moveable room dividers, since if these are disarranged they can easily be restored to order.

Although too often seen, one situation that is to be avoided is illustrated by the following: All the children living on the unit are together in one area, since there is no off-unit activity scheduled at this particular time. The withdrawn children are hovering on chairs or crouching by the walls; the hyperactive ones are running and pacing; some of the more adequate ones may have occupied themselves with a game. The staff members, if they all are there, may be sitting with those few children who are playing, or chatting among themselves. One of the pieces in the game being played may appeal to one of the withdrawn children who comes over to the table and snatches it. The players become angry and aggressive; the child becomes anxious and hyperactive. The staff are now very busy trying to restrain both the players and the child who did the snatching, whereas a little forethought in the shape of appropriate use of time and space, and direct effort to provide activity for the withdrawn children, might have prevented the situation in the first place. The paragraphs that follow contain suggestions on how this planning can be done by the optimally effective use of both human and inanimate resources.

Rest time. Planning rest time is one way in which workers can program. After lunch, instead of milling around aimlessly, the children can be directed to their rooms to rest for a definite amount of time. For the withdrawn children a rest helps to break down time so they know what to expect next. They know that "after lunch we will go into our rooms to rest," and even if they spend the time bouncing on their beds, this is a change of pace for them. The more active children may at first resist such an arrangement. If they are allowed to pursue quiet individual activities on their beds, they may develop the ability to enjoy being and doing things alone. When first introduced to the idea of programming, some child care workers maintain that they do not have sufficient time to organize activities with all the other things they have to do. Instituting a rest period requires no materials and no elaborate planning; it can be built right into the daily life of the children. When a rest time has been successful in a unit program, child care workers find that they enjoy the chance to relax away from the children and to gather their own resources so that they can really be available to the children when they are up. One worker is usually required at rest time to check on and be available to the children in their rooms.

Snack time. Instituting a planned snack period is another method of effectively organizing the program. Most institutions make provisions for juice and crackers or similar snacks to be served between meals. One way of doing this is to hand out the food haphazardly as the children zip by. A more satisfactory way is to build a planned snack time into the program. The children can be encouraged to move the furniture so they have a table surrounded by enough chairs, to serve themselves, and to clean up afterward. While actually eating, the children have a pleasant opportunity to talk together or just be together. Or as in smaller centers, the adults can use the children's time at the table to talk about plans for the rest of the day or to talk about activities that the children have done together. Thus the serving of snacks can become a discrete and meaningful part of the daily program that serves a therapeutic function by breaking down time and space and creating a structure that encourages new learning and more appropriate behavior. Again, this type of plan for serving snacks involves no lengthy planning or coordination.

Clean up. A task which must be done on any unit where there are children is picking and straightening up. Often, however, this job is either done entirely by harried staff or made the responsi-

bility of the oldest, most adequate children, who see it mostly as
an unpleasant chore characteristic of institutionalization. The
picking up may be done before a change of shifts, when the on-
duty shift, to prevent friction from developing, tries to leave
things neat before the next one comes on, as well as at such
routine times as before bed. What is unfortunate about many
cleanup experiences is that the opportunities are ignored to create
another learning experience for many of the younger, more passive children. If a real cleanup time were established and the
younger children were helped to participate in performing real
duties, this routine work of the unit could become therapeutic, in
structuring time and space, increasing expectation, and developing skills. In particular, the fact that the withdrawn children must
really look at their surroundings while picking up makes this
task a valuable type of activity, for the increased aquaintance
they make with the world around them is developing their spatial
orientation. Even the most passive children can learn, if they are
patiently encouraged over a period of time, to pick up papers,
wipe tables, throw scraps in the wastebasket, place pieces of toys
in their boxes, etc. Granted, to involve the less competent children makes the task more time-consuming at first, but the extra
time can be compensated by terminating the previous activity
earlier and by shortening the period of waiting for whatever
comes next, a meal, for example. The effort involved in teaching
the children to help will more than pay off in time.

Daily grooming and care. All the children have to be cared
for physically. At least some aspects of this task can be handled
in such a way that it is a real part of the program defining time
and space. Frequently everything is done for the withdrawn
children—their teeth are brushed for them, their hair is brushed
for them. As was emphasized in a previous chapter, if the time
devoted to such care were instead geared toward teaching the
children to do these things themselves, they would be helped to
develop increased awareness of their own bodies (an important
part of ego development which is usually greatly deficient in the
emotionally disturbed) and some sense of mastery over their

bodies. A beneficial by-product of the self-care program is the development within the children of the feeling that the staff really care about their physical well-being. Verbal children may grumble at first at this routine, but with some of these children nobody ever cared much before how they looked and most of them will come to appreciate the workers' concern. Jay, an angry adolescent from a deprived and chaotic background, would grumble about "mean old Miss Ames," the unit supervisor who made him comb his hair before leaving for school. But within a few months he had acquired a comb of his own which he used frequently. One often hears even normal children say, "Oh, my mother *made* me wear this jacket," but can sense the feeling of pleasure beneath the statement—the pleasure that someone cares enough about them to make them do something.

On-Unit Activity Programming

Even after the scheduled routines have been completed on a unit, there are probably many free hours left when the children are awake and active. Thus it devolves upon the child care worker to plan and organize appropriate activities for his charges —activities that will have appeal, meaning, and applicability to a group that is possibly varied in age, interests, and functioning.

Effective activity programming is so crucial in the care of children that it is useful even in settings that have not yet begun the changeover from custodial to therapeutic care or in institutions which are by their mission custodial. In one institution which housed delinquents who were being held until their cases were disposed of by the court, the staff discovered that the school-age youngsters were very enthusiastic "workers" as long as there was a structured activity in progress. These children, who in civilian life had set fire to houses, thrown rocks at cars, beat up their siblings, etc., were seemingly happy and were very little trouble to manage as long as the staff made a point of letting them be productive. Painting by Numbers was, for instance, a favorite activity. Designing a mural and letting the children paint it was equally successful. At the very least, such a program helps the children to maintain what ego strength they have. They do not deteriorate while they are in "cold storage" waiting for disposal of their cases.

The skeptical worker may be saying to himself at this point, "Well, these ideas about program may have some value, but what can we do with practically no materials in our long corridors?" The clever child care worker can find surprisingly many ways to utilize for program purposes the types of equipment and supplies almost always available in an institution, and he can gain satisfaction from meeting the challenge. For example, chairs and tables can be placed strategically to encourage behavior appropriate to the type of program being offered. A room with chairs arranged around the edges encourages withdrawn children to sit near the walls and active ones to dash around the empty center space. However, a group of chairs arranged in a circle or semicircle makes it easy to start an enjoyable and therapeutic activity of circle games, storytelling, or perhaps just sitting together and conversing. In addition, chairs may be set up as an obstacle course for the children to run (this activity helps to improve their ability to handle their bodies), may be used for games of musical chairs, etc. When a sit-down type of activity is planned, children can help set up the tables and chairs in the kind of arrangement that will invite interest and participation.

When asked, "What do you do on your living area in your spare time?" verbal institutionalized children often say, "Oh, just watch TV." These youngsters are referring to the ubiquitous television set, present and often running constantly on the unit, no matter what the interests, needs, and capabilities of those living there are. One may see withdrawn children wandering around aimlessly while the television buzzes and rattles in the background, ignored by all. Other children may sit lackadaisically in front of the set for hour after hour. This is not to say that there should not be TV sets on children's units. It is to say that the constant, unbroken sound of the television and, for the children who actually watch, the sometimes frightening events on the screen constitute a gross misuse of what could be a therapeutic tool in the child care worker's bag of tricks, serving as another practical application of time-space structure.

First of all, selectivity in programs must be employed. Staff can examine the weekly program guide and pick out those programs which might be suitable for disturbed children to watch. The rest of the time the set must be turned off. For the more withdrawn children, these TV breaks change the pattern of stimulation and provide them with another means of orientation. One way in which withdrawn children learn most effectively is through observation. Appropriate television programs make positive use of this strength. The more active, verbal children can watch programs that are legitimately enjoyable and provide some opportunity for vicarious drain-off of feelings, but do not expose them to more violence or sadistic fantasy than their egos can handle. They can learn about the world from suitable educational programs. The children can learn fitting behavior for quiet activities while watching TV—sitting down, not annoying others, looking at the screen, etc. The TV can even provide a means of helping the worker use himself therapeutically with the group. He can watch some programs along with the children, reassuring them about frightening or unrealistic scenes they may see, explaining what is taking place in the program if necessary, and in general talking with the children about the program. If a busy worker *occasionally* uses the TV to "babysit" the group, he is not necessarily wrong, but he should remember the surprising therapeutic potential of the set.

Let us move from the area of furniture to that of supplies in program improvisation and implementation. The enterprising child care worker can assemble numerous items from routine institutional stock or throwaways that can serve a programming purpose. Maintenance and receiving departments can be asked to save, for example, Styrofoam packing material (which is fun to throw or to use to make collages, decorations, or jewelry) and empty packing boxes and cases (which have endless possibilities —children can crawl in, out, and even on top of them; they can stack them; they can put several together to make houses and trains; aggressive children may be given them to kick and stamp on as acceptable, harmless, and inexpensive outlets).

From the kitchen, workers can get paper plates, with endless possibilities for making decorations, musical instruments, etc. Egg-carton liners can be painted and serve as storage containers. Old tin cans can be decorated to be used for storage and for musical instruments. A nurse may be persuaded to give the workers a box or two of tongue depressors. With glue, or even without, these offer endless construction possibilities for all the children.

From the soft-drink machines in the canteen, bottle caps may be retrieved. The younger children enjoy rummaging through them; the older ones can make buttons and other things from them. All of us probably remember from our own childhoods taking the cork out of a bottle cap, putting the cap on our shirt, and pushing the cork back in on the inside to make it stay on. It is just this sort of experience that many institutionalized children have never had. Seasoned institutional child care workers, understanding the value and need for activity program in the children's lives, probably have many other ideas of how to utilize regular institutional resources. Those suggested here are just a few examples to indicate the possibilities.

What kind of organized activity can possibly be held in the long corridor? Frisbee games, Keep Away (or Monkey in the Middle), roller-skating, mat-tumbling, hopscotch, bowling, ring toss, and relay races—to name just a few—are activities appropriate to this type of space.

Some workers complain that children, particularly the hyperactive ones, destroy anything placed out without direct supervision, which the workers cannot always give when they may be responsible alone for the entire group. This may well be true, and many workers find it wise to store the best materials in a locked cupboard near the children's play area, to be brought out when special supervision is assured. But the children do need materials to have in their hands. Many children, including the most withdrawn ones, enjoy looking at magazines and cutting out pictures with safe blunt scissors. Workers can keep a good bowling set put away for special times and provide ten old plastic detergent bottles for general use. Large plastic toys, such as balls and frisbees, are sturdy and hard to harm or to have do harm. Boxes, cartons, bottle caps, and tongue depressors are also safe and dispensable to be left out for general play.

Grouping

Although a volume could be written on the art of group composition and group management of children, there are a few key points of grouping that are related to the effectiveness of the total program. One of the basic points is that of the child care worker's responsibility for the physical safety of the children in his care. This means that he must know where the children are at all times, and it is necessary that some children be within the worker's sight at all times. While it certainly is understood that there are many demands on the child care worker's time, such as clothing maintenance, housekeeping tasks that the children cannot do even with help, and report writing, and that there are times from the point of view of the program when there just is not enough supervision to allow certain activities to take place, *for reason of both physical safety and sound psychological practice, at least one worker must always be present in the area where the children are.* It takes only a few minutes for a tragedy to occur among unsupervised children. The possibility of such an occurrence increases, too, whenever there are knots of all the on-duty workers chatting among themselves or working together in an area closed off from the children.

If the worker in charge of the group has work to do, he can often do much of it with the children. For example, if he has clothing to fold, he can take this into the area where the children are and chat with some of them or even have them help him do the job. This practice is much sounder from the therapeutic point of view also. The children themselves need to know that there is an adult near by, even though he may not be able to "do anything" with them right now. And it is good for them to see the adult taking care of their clothing, rather than to have it reappear magically in their dresser drawers. However, at the same time when administrators insist that there should always be on-the-spot supervision of children, they should also be sure that every child care worker has short times to be away from the children completely. It is well worth the effort to *insist* that every worker take at least two breaks per tour of duty in addition to his meal break and to make arrangements so that this can take place.

The alert child care worker tries to see how he can help the children in the group to use each other therapeutically. This point does not, of course, mean that certain children are put in charge of the rest of the group while the adults busy themselves elsewhere. The errors in this practice hardly need to be mentioned; a major one is, of course, the fact that this kind of authority is too tempting to the weak egos and controls of the children in charge and frightening to the younger children. However, by ingenious grouping and subgrouping, patterns of interacting can be encouraged that are growth-producing in the children and incidentally helpful to shorthanded staff in helping them to stretch themselves further. For example, on walks the older children can, under the supervision of the staff, hold the hands of the younger children who otherwise might stray from the group, thus providing a valid way for the older children to be helpful and a sensible type of contact for the younger ones. The same kind of arrangement can be implemented for some other activities, although at times the children like to be free to mingle informally among themselves.

Another suitable way for both withdrawn and active children to relate constructively to one another is for the older ones to read to the younger ones. Although this activity might have to be handled with tact and special consideration, since many of the active children are aware that they cannot read as well as others their age, it is ego-building for those children who have mastered some reading skills in intramural school, in addition to providing a suitable activity for the others who listen. At times, the worker may feel that there are certain children who would be helped through a relationship with certain other children. The worker can promote this friendship by having them work on a project or task together, thus providing a basis for developing a relationship. (For further discussion see the section "Caring for Other Children" in chapter 9.)

At times when all the child care staff can be with the children, it is often more effective and therapeutic if the children can be divided into small groups for activities appropriate to each one and, if possible, go to separate areas. This permits closer supervision and interaction to take place. For example, one might see one child care worker in a room with the more withdrawn children listening to music and playing a circle game, while in a second room another worker may be helping the more reality-focused children set up and play a table game.

Special Events

An amazingly successful way of bringing out through group activity the potentialities of both staff and children is through the special event. Child care workers on institutional units sometimes complain of being in a rut. Planning and executing some type of program different from what is done every day sometimes serve to unify and challenge the staff. Workers find themselves looking at the children differently as the children rise toward the new expectations offered through the new activity. In planning a play, for example, the staff must get together to decide how and when it will be given, what parts the children can take, what materials will be needed, how to give the children as much responsibility and opportunity to participate as possible, etc. The enthusiasm which they often generate is then communicated to the children, resulting often in more purposeful and appropriate behavior than has ever been seen. This gratification often renews the staff members' faith in themselves and in the rehabilitative potential of their charges. Many institutions hold open houses to which parents or various members of the public are invited to see the children's facilities and program. Although sometimes from the legal and always from the psychological point of view care has to be taken in exposing the children to observers, these kinds of programs can be therapeutic if executed well, with planning and regard for the particular children involved. The putting on of a skit, the serving of refreshments, the dressing up in best clothing for a legitimate purpose, all are experiences the children may never have had before. These special events help provide the children with a sense of belonging, of being more like normal children, of mastery, of acceptability to other people, and of having a link with the outside world.

Programming Within the Institutional Structure

The suggestion was made earlier that the many nonclinical departments of the large institution (those not involved in direct service to children) can be an asset as well as a liability in work with disturbed children. Workers in many of the departments which maintain the day-to-day life of the institution are often quite interested in the children and will cooperate in giving them special attention if this does not interfere too greatly with their work. By arrangement with various departments, children can be taken on trips to the kitchen to see how their food is cooked, to the laundry to see how their clothes are washed, to the various shops to see how equipment is repaired, etc. Sometimes a maintenance worker may have time and inclination to give a few lessons in carpentry to some of the bigger boys. If such close cooperation with other departments is forthcoming, child care workers have an obligation to see that when the children make their visits, they are not destructive and do not become a nuisance to other workers, who after all have their own tasks to accomplish.

Members of other departments have certain necessary contacts with the children in the course of daily living. If the child care workers feel that the performance or the attitude of a member of some other department is not in the best interests of the children, they can sometimes get improvement if they make their feelings known through appropriate channels.

In one children's unit within an adult hospital, meals were brought up and served by any one of several dietary workers. One of these workers found the children's mealtime behavior very discomfiting and sometimes handed out the food with angry remarks to the youngsters. The workers, who of course had expectations for more socialized behavior at meals but who were adjusting and timing their efforts to the needs of individual children, were greatly distressed at the attitude of this particular dietary worker, and they conveyed their distress to the unit supervisor. He in turn started negotiations with the dietary department to try to have a regular person bring the food for each meal—one who by temperament could be sympathetic to the workers' efforts with the children. The negotiations took several months, but in the end his request was fulfilled, with the result that the mealtime atmosphere was far more therapeutic.

In another institution where the constant requests for repairs to toys and equipment had become a nuisance to the maintenance department, a small repair shop was started on the unit with one of the child care workers in charge and with the maintenance department furnishing advice and scraps of lumber and the like for the unit. This reorganization not only improved relations with the maintenance department but was of great benefit to the children. On the same unit it was found to be possible for some of the better-controlled children to stay and watch when a major repair of some sort was in progress, rather than for all to be cleared off the unit, as had previously been necessary.

A judicious effort by child care workers to build and maintain positive relationships with nonclinical as well as clinical staff usually benefits all concerned. The interest generated in the children by the nonclinical staff helps to increase the resources available to the children and helps to broaden the scope of their contacts with different people.

CHAPTER 8

The Worker and Institutional Policies: Discipline

Chapter 7 describes an approach to overall programming by the child care worker in the institution, with reference both to daily living and to activities on the living unit. In addition to this large portion of his daily work, however, the child care worker is frequently confronted with difficult situations and behavior about which he may have to make a decision, often right on the spot. It helps greatly if the worker understands many aspects of institutional policy, operation, and philosophy; he has to apply these in many practical situations.

All institutions have certain policies, rules governing the handling of a wide variety of situations and behaviors. Some policies may be realistic and effective; others may be rigid and difficult to comply with and accept. The worker may well encounter some policies with which he does not agree and which he is tempted not to obey. This chapter discusses some types of policies the worker is likely to encounter in the large institution and some of the background thinking that may have been involved in setting them up. It also describes what the worker's relationship to these policies might be, so that ultimately whatever he does is of greatest benefit to the children and thus of greatest satisfaction to him.

One of the broadest, most crucial, and most controversial issues in institutional child care is that of discipline. There is no setting for children, it would seem, where the practices and attitudes concerning discipline are not the subject of frequent, sometimes heated discussion among the staff. The area of discipline has two aspects, one which is concerned with the background issues and one which deals with practical and specific applications. While the child care worker may be most directly involved with the latter, the nature of his work would, for him to serve most effectively, necessitate his familiarity with the former.

Definition

A working definition of the term *discipline* is essential to any basic consideration of the subject, since often the term discipline is confused with *punishment*. One frequently hears it said, for example, that children must be disciplined for committing some offense, when really what the speaker means is that the children should be punished. *Punishment,* in the strictest sense of the word, is a specific negative act performed as a response to another act which is negative in the eyes of the punisher and which he does not want to have repeated. The term *discipline,* however, has a broader and more positive meaning, one which is related to overall child development and to achievement of happy and constructive living. Discipline is considered as a positive encouragement, guidance, and teaching of the kind of behavior which helps a child to learn to live as a socialized being and to achieve the optimum growth and development which is possible for him. This type of discipline is not achieved by frequent use of punitive practices and highly restrictive controls, applied as a direct consequence of some disapproved specific action on the part of the children. Rather, it is built into every aspect of an institutional program and supported by concentrated efforts of the staff to sustain relevant points of view, practices, and policies.

Looking for Reasons

Staff in an institution attempting to promote positive discipline try to look beyond the immediate disturbing behavior for possible causes, which can then be altered if necessary or at least worked through with the children involved. For example, if a child runs away from the institution, the staff could, on the child's return, apply immediate and decisive punitive measures such as isolation and deprivation. These actions taken solely would only serve to increase the child's negative feelings, which probably made him want to run away in the first place, toward the institution. On the other hand, if the staff attempt to find out why he ran away and help correct, or help him correct, the reasons underlying the behavior, the experience can be one of true learning. Other disciplinary practices are more humane if applied in a context of helping the child come to grips with the feelings and situations related to his running away. Although this is just one example, the child care worker should bear in mind that in his daily work he has many opportunities for handling similar situations and that each one has the possibility of helping the child learn in a way that will be one step toward, not away from, health.

This is not to say, of course, that for every episode of disturbed behavior the child care worker must conduct a profound search into possible causes. From the point of view of time this is not always feasible. For many things that happen during the day, often the immediate goal is to help the child get calm so that he can rejoin the program without additional probing on the worker's part. However, it is definitely the role of any child care worker to hold a point of view about discipline, and in this sense the worker needs to know the part that reasons play in misbehavior and their relation to punishment.

Prevention

Another key element in a philosophy of institutional discipline is prevention. The child care worker can help to create a climate on the living unit in which incidents that staff members are tempted to handle by punishment are less likely to occur; such a climate is one which also helps the children to grow. Preventive discipline, then, involves setting up the environment in such a way that it encourages and allows the children to behave in a constructive and growth-producing way and holds out expectations that they are capable of meeting. It is closely related to the general principles of therapeutic programming described in chapter 7, for children are less likely to get into mischief if they have enough to do.

To give an example of preventive discipline in everyday family life, mothers know that there are certain children with whom their own offspring can play peacefully and constructively for just a certain amount of time before they begin to overstimulate one another. To avoid having a pitched battle to referee, with unhappy feelings all around, the mother plans these contacts to end before trouble starts and she is required to assume a negative role. This aspect of child care has many parallels in an institution. For preventive discipline the children are not exposed to, or left to their own devices in, any situation involving an activity, a group, or a routine for a time longer than they can cope with.

The workers' use of the time-space concept takes on new meaning here. Preventive discipline must always take time into account. It involves planning activities for only the amount of time that the children can participate effectively or stopping group interaction or activities at a point before they disintegrate. Seasoned child care workers become skilled at this. They seem to know when a half hour TV program, carefully selected, will be more beneficial to the group than a two-hour movie, which, after an hour has passed, will have most of the group wiggling in their seats and hissing at one another; they seem to know just when to tell the group in the midst of a pillow fight, "Okay, let's taper off now so we can have our snack," before real anger and bedlam set in. By using the factor of timing in managing the children, then, the worker can prevent many unpleasant and difficult situations from arising.

Space and its uses must also be kept in mind in preventive discipline. Staff must consider not only how space is subdivided but also how materials and activities are designed to utilize this space effectively.

In an institution of active disturbed adolescent boys, the main space available on the living unit was a large one, furnished mainly by chairs which lined the wall, a few tables, and a television set. The staff caring for the youngsters had frequent difficulty with fights, destruction, and rule-breaking, as the boys mingled in the large room. All the staff of the institution debated how to solve the problem of the boys' behavior; some talked about the necessity of punishment such as isolation and deprivation of program. As a positive approach activity workers were assigned to go on the unit at "in-between" times, when the boys were neither in school nor at meals or other scheduled events. Supplies of craft and game material were made available; the workers were instructed to subdivide the boys into small groups, rearranging tables and chairs in order to create an inviting setting and to establish physical limits for the group activity. Each group was to be involved in an activity which would be of interest to the individuals. After a week or so, a distinct change was noticed in the behavior of the boys. Destruction, aggression, and acting-out behavior took place much less frequently, and such conduct had a more rational basis when it did occur. The boys, many of whom had an impoverished background of experiences, not only were easier for the staff to manage from a practical point of view, but were enjoying and profiting from the ego-building activities which they had not previously been exposed to. With the change in the group behavior, encouraged by rearranging the space and program of the unit, there was considerably less talk about the need for stricter measures to be taken.

In short, a carefully planned environment, which allows and encourages constructive behavior, increases the children's sense of security, mastery, and well-being. It counteracts boredom, hyperactivity, and aggression and serves as an effective agent for preventive discipline.

Discipline at the Developmental Level

Discipline at the developmental level is the expectation and tolerance of behavior at the individual child's or the group's level of maturity—at a place where he or they can be expected to be capable of performing or conforming. It also involves recognition of behavior which would normally be characteristic of children's behavior at earlier ages, that is, recognizing when a child is acting younger than he really is. In these areas a worker's knowledge of basic development and deviation from basic development is most helpful.

The worker's understanding of the fact that most school-age children find meaning in "junk" collections will help him temper his aggravation at what he finds in Johnny's bureau drawer with awareness that such hoarding is the way with children of his age. Understanding the importance of grooming fads to teen-agers will help the worker tolerate—if not promote—these in his group and not make an unnecessary issue over them. Realizing that young children, especially some disturbed ones, cannot sit still long can guide the worker to avoid including these children in situations where they must be still for too long a time. There are many other examples in institutional life where a knowledge of basic development can help the worker guide the children constructively and avoid causing issues and situations in which the children's behavior would possibly result in negative consequences.

Discipline and Freedom

The nature and amount of freedom granted to institutionalized children are important issues in the overall area of discipline. Participation in decisions on such matters can be one of the most difficult aspects of the child care worker's job. Some workers may feel that freedom to roam the grounds at will, have money to spend freely, mingle with the opposite sex, and choose whether or not to participate in activities is appropriate and reasonable for all. Others may feel that the children need to be closely controlled and guarded, that they should proceed quietly from area to area in line and display "refined" language and deportment at all times. Fortunately, most child care workers fall between these extremes, and it also seems that a compromise between these two approaches offers the most reasonable practice. In institutional living one would want to avoid both overregimentation and total disorder; in other words, children may be granted various freedoms in increasing degree as they demonstrate their ability to handle them.

Schoolteachers often comment that they start out the year with "strict" control and gradually ease up, rather than allowing too much freedom at first and having the more difficult task of clamping down later. In the institution, as an example, the children should not be allowed extensive ground privileges at first and then be completely restricted when they show that they cannot handle them yet. Rather, either as a group or as individuals, they should be allowed increasing access to off-unit areas as they demonstrate their ability to handle this freedom. The first step might be to release them to specific appointments with passes; the second, to appointments without passes; the third, to limited free time to go to certain areas on the grounds; the fourth, to longer free-time periods within a greater area, etc. At each step the child or group indicates its ability to handle the next one.

The granting of freedom can be regulated to the individual needs and disturbances of the children. A girl whose "problem" is promiscuous sexual behavior would not be allowed to have access without supervision to areas where boys are present. A boy whose difficulties include illicit smoking would be prevented from having access to areas where cigarettes are available until he can withstand the temptation of such exposure. A child who flies off the handle when things get too noisy would when possible be kept away from areas where there is confusing hustle and bustle until he is better oriented.

Workers may be asking at this point how gradual granting of freedom is related to discipline. When there is overrestriction, with no way for children to aspire to increasing independence and its associated pleasures, they become resentful and angry and seek the first opportunity to "get around" the adults. As the adults perceive these attitudes, they tighten the rein even more, and a vicious circle develops in which the adults are punitive and the children spend all their energy trying to outwit them and stand up to their punishments. In this situation, they certainly are not learning or developing in a positive way. However, when there is not *enough* control or planning of the experiences that the children are exposed to, their symptoms and undeveloped controls may cause them to behave in ways disturbing to the staff and harmful to themselves, possibly also resulting in punishment. To illustrate, during a time when the boy with the smoking problem is free to roam without supervision, he takes money from a staff member's pocketbook and buys cigarettes from the staff machine. What are the results? First of all, the staff are angry. The feelings of staff from other units may also be involved; they may say, "Those kids sure have the run of this place" or "They can sure get away with anything." Actually, this latter statement is probably not the case. The general disgruntlement results in a punishment which makes the miscreant feel angry and revengeful and only increases the probability of future wrongdoing. Had the boy been prevented access to these areas at this stage of his treatment, the damaging event might not have occurred.

This concept does not mean that institutionalized children should be deprived of every experience in which there is a possible risk of their behaving inappropriately. It only means that the gains should be weighed against the risks. One worker recalls a meeting where several of the workers were disturbed about the symptomatic behavior of the children, especially in off-unit situations. They were reminded that these children *were* disturbed, that their symptomatic behavior was the reason for their admission, and that their behavior much of the time was going to reflect this, but that they needed the exposure to different situations in order to get better. While the program should not *overexpose* the children to more than they can cope with, at the same time it must not shield them from all challenge or newness. In fact, for them to grow and to be oriented to the final goal of return to the community, some challenge is necessary. The children must come to know the world outside the institution; at the same time they must have an opportunity to express their feelings about the things they see and hear so that the staff can try to understand and help them with these feelings.

As the children are gradually exposed to new and more challenging experiences, they can be encouraged to control their behavior according to the area and social characteristics of the situation they are in. For example, they can be made to understand that their more colorful language, if they really need to use it, must be saved for the home unit; that if they are to be allowed access to outside areas, they must "save" their desire to talk this way until later. Or a child who needs to, and at times is allowed to, act like a much younger child, may be reminded that such behavior is appropriate and acceptable in a therapy session, but not on a special off-grounds shopping trip. The adolescent girl attached to a pair of faded jeans with nail-polish pictures on them may be allowed to wear them on the unit but must wear a dress to school.

Staff Values and Discipline

Since the attitudes toward discipline differ among staff members in accordance with their personality, background, and training, there is often disagreement among them as to which behavior should be allowed and which forbidden. There are some who think mouths should be washed out with soap for swearing; others who feel it is wisest to ignore foul language. The fact that staff members have different feelings about how behavior should be handled can confuse the children and affect the quality of care unless workers attempt at least to compromise their differences so that they can present a united front to the children. If the staff's disagreement about how different situations should be dealt with is not resolved, feelings of anger toward different members may arise, and they may "act out" their feelings in front of the children. For example a disagreeing worker might say, "Well, I'd certainly like to let you go buy some pop, but Mr. X. says I'm not allowed to" or, "I don't know where your good shoes are—that other shift never keeps the clothing in order." This type of situation is relevant to discipline because it prevents the children from recognizing the constructive authority of the entire staff. If they perceive there is disagreement, they are then unsure of the limits set by different individuals, see no reason to respect the rules, and test the staff even more to see where the real limits are. Dissension also tends to divide the staff into opposite camps, making some seem like kind gratifiers and others like unreasonable scolds; and this again does not promote effective and constructive discipline. Child care workers in disagreement about discipline and limits need to assume a collaborative adult attitude, to establish mutually agreed on objectives and means so that they will put the total welfare of the children before their own wish to have revenge on one another. They must try to reach compatible attitudes so that all can offer consistent guidelines to the children.

Also, the fact that children like a worker is not always a criterion of his effectiveness. Some workers feel that in order to be successful, they must make themselves likable to the children to the extent of not enforcing the rules and limits that have been established as guidelines for them. While children may talk about their dislike for certain policies and for the workers as they enforce them, in the long run the children will not have negative feelings for the workers if they are treated fairly and consistently. As a matter of fact, the children usually respect and learn more from the worker who has the strength of spirit to help them meet those reasonable limits and expectations which serve to improve their social and intellectual performance.

An activities worker with a group of highly impulsive children found this principle illustrated any number of times in his work in crafts with the children. A child would start a project, such as a lanyard, and at the first obstacle or frustration would want to abandon it and start something else. However, the worker would kindly, but firmly, insist that the current project be completed and offer whatever support necessary so that this could be achieved, reminding the children that "the rule is that if you begin something, you need to finish it." The childrens' pride and pleasure at their completed projects—"Look what I *made!*" they would tell their other workers—was evidence that the temporary anger aroused in the children when they were not permitted to start a new project paled in the sense of achievement they received from their finished work.

Not to react to a child's loss of control is nontherapeutic. To react properly can be highly therapeutic. As the ultimate goal is to develop self-discipline in the children—the ability to control their own behavior—so must self-discipline be a characteristic of the worker whose actions serve as a model for the children with whom he works so closely.

The worker may be wondering why so much space has been given in this chapter to the subject of discipline. Although this is a most important aspect of dealing with children in any setting, it takes on additional significance in the institution because there the ratio of children to staff is large, and thus there is a genuine problem of management of the children. The preceding discussion has served as a background survey of the general issue of discipline and punishment, to help the worker form a philosophy of his own and to indicate that there is an important positive aspect to discipline. On the job, however, the child care worker will perhaps encounter a variety of practices designed to control and/or punish the children. The subsequent section discusses and evaluates various aspects of some of these practices.

Institutional Methods of Discipline and Management

Isolation. Unlike many smaller centers, most institutions have isolation rooms—bare, locked rooms in which there is no way for a child to hurt himself or the furnishings. (In some states it is illegal to place a patient behind a locked door without a medical order and a plan for periodic checking.) While there is sometimes controversy about whether such a room should be used at all, it should be kept in mind that many benign settings do have them. Thus it would seem that the most relevant issue is not whether or not there should be such a room, but how it can be used appropriately and hygienically and how it can be misused.

In the first place, when there is enough staff, skillful handling and adequate program can greatly reduce or even eliminate the use of the isolation room. In some centers with an adequate ratio of workers to children, isolation rooms have been completely eliminated as the program and handling have improved, and, conversely, the use of isolation has been introduced in units when the program and quality of care have deteriorated. It must be recognized, however, that if the ratio of children to staff is high, the isolation room is sometimes a necessary resource for children who become so physically upset that they cannot be contained by the staff.

Needless to say, careful consideration should be given to which children are placed there. As a rule of thumb, it is unwise in general to isolate withdrawn children if it is at all possible to do otherwise, for it only reinforces their own tendencies to isolate themselves and it may frighten them. Besides, in their case physically upset behavior is often a sign of improvement. When a withdrawn child who has never before overtly expressed anger hits out at somebody who annoys him, he may be truly progressing, and his action does not warrant punishment by isolation. On the other hand, the isolation of acting-out children, if properly timed, can serve to help them become more reflective about the difficulties which made them upset (and they often cannot become reflective in a more stimulating environment), and it can physically contain them so as to avoid injury and destruction.

A boy in a treatment center would at times become frenzied with anger during activities with the other children. Any attempts on the part of workers to deal with him on the spot would only increase his upset, which would be directed against the workers as well as the other children. After a period of isolation, he would be calm enough so that a trusted worker could trace with him what in the situation had made him so angry and how he might have most effectively handled these feelings. Only in this solitude did it seem possible, for a while anyway, for this child to be able to look beneath the surface of any of his actions.

In essence, then, isolation judiciously used can be helpful, but it has a number of pitfalls also. One of these is keeping children isolated for too long a time—long after they have regained physical control and are behaviorally ready to join the group. For any child too long a period of isolation can approximate a condition of "stimulus deprivation." For psychotic children especially, this situation gives even more opportunity for development of unrealistic thoughts, fears, fantasies of abandonment, and wishes for revenge.

Then acting-out children may feel that the punishment is over-severe and use this as justification of their feelings that adults are mean; and the probability of their acting out again is greatly increased.

When a child is isolated, the staff should use the occasion not only as an act of containment but as an opportunity to talk with him about the situation. Isolation loses its effectiveness when performed mechanically. The children do not respect it and, even more important, certainly do not benefit from it.

It is possible for a child care staff to fall into the trap of using isolation as a punishment for anything and everything, instead of as a necessary resource for a child who has really lost physical control of himself. Workers should watch such threats as, "If you don't listen to me, you're going to the isolation ['quiet,' 'back,' or whatever the institution calls it] room." They should be constantly on the alert to the possibility of overusing and misusing this method of controlling the children, so that what positive value it does have is preserved.

Restriction and deprivation. Deprivation of privileges as a method of control or discipline is also frequently employed in institutions. Children who misbehave or do not do certain things which are expected of them may not be allowed to attend recreational activities, go outside on ground passes, go to a weekly movie, etc. If not used in excess, this does not have to be non-therapeutic. In fact, if misbehavior occurs in a situation or activity that the children like, it is often more appropriate to make some type of deprivation of that particular activity (the amount of time depending on the severity of the offense) than to institute some unrelated measure. There are occasionally specific situations where this type of restriction is indicated, for example, a child who has been returned from school for misbehavior should not be allowed to roam the halls on his ground pass, at least during school hours.

Like isolation, restriction and deprivation of activities have certain pitfalls. There is often friction when child care staff want to deprive a child of another department's activity. If this is to be done, there must be preliminary agreement among all that it is acceptable and on how it is to be done. It is true that some child care workers feel that they are the only ones who do not have many gratifying activities to take away from the children to help control their behavior. These individuals may be heartened by the understanding that activities are not just something which is fun for the children but are an essential part of their treatment and as much a part of their program as therapy sessions. Particularly if the activity diet available to the children is limited and if the children are withdrawn in the first place, activity deprivation can be taking away the very things they need to get better and to be able to behave in a more acceptable way. (See also the discussion of other disciplines under "Staff Relationships" in chapter 11.)

Point systems. Some institutions have point systems whereby children either earn points by good behavior or lose points by bad behavior. If they lose too many points or do not earn enough, depending on how the particular system is set up, they lose some privilege. There is a rigid and unsympathetic aspect to point systems when they do not accommodate to individual treatment needs or symptoms of the children. The main asset of rigid point systems may not be in their effectiveness as treatment tools with the children but in their being a means of encouraging staff communication about the children. Workers will inevitably share experiences and observations while evaluating children to award the points. In an indirect way the children may benefit because the system has helped the staff to consolidate their practices and points of view.

It goes without saying that in any rigid and automatic point system, the liabilities outweigh the assets. It is possible, however, to set up a more discriminating kind of point system which may be both productive and therapeutic. Certain key principles must be kept in mind. In the first place, the system cannot be applied to the whole living situation of the children—this is too complicated and thus impractical. It can be best applied to the classroom, to work tasks, or to any other highly structured segment of the child's life. Secondly, a point system must be so structured as to involve rewards and not deprivations, that is, the extension of privileges which the children are ready for and not the restriction of activities which they need as part of their treatment. Set up in this fashion, a point system simply formalizes something that the staff look at anyway, when they examine the behavior of individuals to determine whether they are ready for new privileges; it is a way in which the staff can communicate the decision process to the children. A third principle is that such a point system is applicable only to those children who can understand its use and meaning; it is not applicable to withdrawn children.

In other words, if a point system is generated out of the needs of the staff, as a control mechanism, it is bound to fail. It breaks down and becomes a punishment system, detrimental to the children's welfare, and not a reward system. If it is generated out of the needs of the youngsters who are capable of understanding what it is all about, offering them landmarks by which to measure their own progress, it can be very useful.

Ward meeting. Some institutions include in their program a system of meetings in which children can discuss various aspects of their lives in the institution. Properly designed and executed, such a regular meeting can be of great value in promoting a structured dialogue between the staff and the children, in which much information is conveyed to the staff about the success of their own planning and the execution of their plans. Matters that should be corrected can often be pointed out by the children, and all protests should be carefully examined, no matter how unreasonable they may seem. The children may also be permitted to make certain decisions which affect their lives and which are within their competence, and this freedom can be of great value in helping them to achieve independence and in counteracting their tendency to become institutionalized.

The ward discussion can, however, become detrimental if it is utilized as a means of having peers determine the penalties for other children who misbehave (Individual children may sometimes assess their own penalties, but that is another matter.) To allow children to assess one another's penalties reinforces the natural tyranny of children, particularly of disturbed ones who may have severely impaired judgment and poor impulse control, and makes more likely the occurrence of "kangaroo courts" when the adults are not present, with resulting cruel and unusual punishments. It is the responsibility of the adults to correct any misbehavior of the children, and this responsibility cannot be delegated to the youngsters; this rule makes group life safer and more secure for all.

Extra work. Extra work assignments are sometimes used as punishments for children who break an institution's rules. In addition to everyday chores which the children are expected to perform, a child may be asked to do yard, kitchen, janitorial, or other work as a penalty. In some institutions miscreants are given as punishment useless "busy work," such as pushing a dry mop around a floor and cutting grass with scissors. This practice is of dubious value, to say the most for it, since it is highly undignified and overpunitive if required for any but the briefest time.

Required work can be meaningful and instructive when it is related to what the child did. For example, if a child has written on walls, it is logical for him to be required to scrub off the writing. If a child has stolen money, it is reasonable for him to work to repay it by, for example, washing cars or shining shoes. Some child care workers feel that having children do extra work as a penalty for breaking rules interferes with the therapeutic goal of the child's learning to value his own productivity by reinforcing negative attitudes toward work. There is merit to this belief. On the other hand, it would seem that a modest additional and appropriate work assignment can show a child that his actions are not being ignored and that he is expected to make restitution; and this process can be constructive.

Corporal punishment. It goes without saying that corporal punishment would be forbidden in any institution which espouses any kind of humane care. Usually it is forbidden by law or institutional policy. However, occasionally there is a staff member who feels that such punishment is the only way of controlling the children. "All he needs to keep him in line is a good spanking" is the way one sometimes hears this sentiment expressed, or, "I've tried everything else!" The disadvantages of such a practice do not have to be elaborated; rather it should be emphasized that there are many more effective alternatives open to the worker.

A distinction should be clear to the child care worker between physical punishment and physical control in the form of holding or physically moving a child. Some children have episodes of very upset behavior in which the worker finds that they must be restrained to prevent injury to themselves, others, or furnishings. The worker may have to hold the child to contain his activity until he regains control of himself. When a worker is thus trying to control a child, the child often interprets the worker's behavior as punitive. The worker can verbalize to the child what he is doing, for example, "I'm holding you until you feel more calm." It is important then that the worker be very sure of what he is doing and maintain his own control, so that the child does not manipulate him into actually being punitive. He must be careful not to be covertly punitive, not to hold too tightly or to jerk the child.

An angry child may continually try to hit a staff member, to the point where it is necessary for the worker to hold the child's hands until he is able to calm down. This restraint involves no physical punishment of the child, as would the staff member's hitting him back. Or a small child may suddenly plop down on the floor when it is time for his group to go to another area. The worker may have to go over to him and while gently talking to him, also lift him up and move him along to join the rest of the group. This is not physical punishment, although it would have been had the child been angrily dragged and pushed along.

Verbal control. Verbal methods of course are the most frequently used means of controlling and managing children and usually are the first resort when a worker feels that some piece of behavior must be rechannelled. These can be used in both a positive and a negative fashion. Often the greatest difference in approach to the children observed in staff members is the way in which they talk to the children and what they say. The basic goodwill of the worker and his liking for children necessarily come through as he talks to them. True enough, a busy child care worker responsible for a large number of children may find himself occasionally exasperated and once in a while responding more abruptly or angrily than he wishes. This lapse will not hurt the children if they feel sure that basically he likes them.

One worker whose manner with the children was usually mild and easygoing finally verbally lost his temper with the children one day when there had been one incident of wild behavior after another. The last straw came when, shouting loudly, the boys were running up and down the hall swatting at the overhead lights with wet towels. The worker suddenly shouted, "You kids better get out of the hall and into the living room in two seconds flat—and I don't want to hear another word out of you either!" The children, never having heard the worker raise his voice before, were so surprised that they quickly and meekly complied.

This example is given not to suggest that such outbursts should take place on a frequent basis, but simply to point out that within the context of a positive relationship, a worker's showing his human feelings does not have to be harmful. Later, both worker and children can sometimes share the humor in such situations. One who finds himself reacting like this frequently, however, needs to reexamine his attitudes and practices. Nobody with any kind of therapeutic intentions would practice or support loud, enraged scolding or yelling, biting sarcasm and humiliation, or chronic "crabbiness" which can be not only harmful to the children but destructive to staff morale and relationships. These techniques are not practiced by successful child care workers.

The way in which the individual child care worker handles the children's misbehavior is determined in part by institutional policies and the prevalent approach of the entire staff as they implement these policies in day-to-day living, as well as by his own attitudes and personality. These are at times in conflict. In some situations the worker will have to compromise between what he thinks is best and what accepted practice demands. Occasionally he may feel unable to compromise, if he believes that what is being done to a child is truly harmful. One would hope that he would have access to at least one person on the institution's supervisory and/or administrative staff with whom he could discuss his feelings and the reasons for them and with whom he could plan a constructive approach to dealing with the situation.

The institutional child care worker's stand for positive discipline based on his understanding of children and the use of his child care skills to promote this stand, both directly and indirectly, are among the greatest contributions he can make to the forward growth of the children in his care.

CHAPTER 9

The Worker and Institutional Policies: Relationships and Related Matters

The discussion of institutional policy toward discipline has placed the topic of discipline within a broader framework, since the concept of discipline is so deeply relevant to the function of the child care worker and to the therapeutic care of the children. There are other aspects of institutional policy and practices which have similar implications.

Medication

Many child care programs today use medication as part of their therapeutic endeavor. Since, of course, medication is used to alter behavior and also may have physical side effects on the children, discussion of the relationship of medication to child care work is germane here. In some settings the child care workers, under the supervision of a nurse, are responsible for the administration of medication, and it is, therefore, also helpful for the workers to be aware of various attitudes and reactions the children might have to the actual administering process.

The child care worker will be interested in the overall philosophy of the institution on the use of medication, as well as in the effects of a specific prescription on a given child's behavior. Since the medical staff, of course, are responsible for these aspects of the program, they are the ones from whom this information would be obtained.

Some workers dislike the idea of the children's receiving any medication; others may feel that medication should be the first and automatic answer to any behavior or management problem. The worker can consider the following: medication can make many children more amenable to the program and to the relationship offered by the worker. Hyperactive children may become stable and controlled; withdrawn children may become more interested and involved with the surrounding environment. Of course, if medication were used indiscriminately in massive doses to sedate the children so that they were never any trouble, it would be a misuse of what otherwise is an important treatment tool. When medication helps the children to become more open to the benefits of a treatment program, it is a positive aspect of that program; if it were used to the extent that the children never had the opportunity to work through difficult situations, the opposite would be the case.

An example of the positive use of medication in an institutional setting is the case of a child who very much needed gratifying experiences but who almost always became upset before such experiences were to take place. He would try to provoke the adults around him into denying him a pleasant event, such as a trip to a farm, and thus confirm his feelings that they were mean and stingy. In reality the child was not in condition to leave the residence when he was so upset; and although isolation would ultimately help him calm down, it took a long time to do so, and, of course, he would miss the important trip. This therapeutic dilemma was handled by the psychiatrist's giving the child a tranquilizing injection when he got upset, and by the time the group was actually ready to leave he was calm and ready too and thus able to enjoy some of the benefits the trip had for him. Eventually the staff needed to watch for the time when it would be most therapeutic for him to learn to cope without the extra aid of medication with his feelings about special experiences and the adults that could offer them.

The child care worker administering medication under medical supervision may encounter various responses, such as fear, grogginess, and reduced appetite. Some children are frightened at the prospect of swallowing a mysterious substance and need explanation and reassurance: "We hope this will make you feel more like doing things"; "This will help you control yourself"; "This is a capsule with some medicine in it that will make you feel better."

Whether or not the worker is administering medication, he needs to learn from the medical staff what the side effects of the medicine may be. The worker who realizes that a reduced appetite is an expected side effect of a certain drug will take this into account at mealtime and not become alarmed when the child eats less than usual. The worker who knows that a medicine may make a child feel groggy will allow a little more time for getting up from a rest and into the daily routine. When he knows that certain tranquilizers make people more susceptible to sunburn, he can see that children are protected by hats, lotions, or shade.

Presents and Treats

Many institutions have policies concerning giving to children; frequently the rule is that no staff member is permitted to give gifts to individual children. Workers who are aware of the apparent need of a child for some material gratifications and who themselves very much want to give to the children sometimes find this policy hard to abide by. A specific example may illustrate the thinking behind such a policy:

One day Joan, a child care worker, brought in a new blouse for Marie, one of the girls she particularly liked. Marie told her roommate how she had gotten it and of course the roommate wanted one too. She asked Joan to get her one, and Joan, wanting to stay in the good graces of the children, got her one too. Before Joan knew it, she was being asked by all the children to buy them things.

This incident points up some of the pitfalls of individual giving: one is that other children may feel the worker is showing favoritism and likes the child receiving the gift the most; another is that the worker can get into a situation which can be overtaxing financially or may jeopardize his relationships with the children if he tries to stop.

Another aspect of giving found in large institutions is the tendency of the institution—and interested community organizations with the permission of the institution—to shower the children with parties and presents at certain holiday times and to ignore them the rest of the year. Related to this is the interest of some staff members in developing intense relationships with a certain few children so that they want to take them home for visits with their own families. On the surface, both of these things seem like benign and generous activities, and this is certainly their intention. But the staff, in planning special experiences, relationships, and treats, should keep in mind various aspects of the institutional experience so as to assure that the children's needs are really appropriately met. Children in institutions, like children at home, can get a surfeit of parties and treats if too many are offered in rapid succession, especially if these require only passive participation.

In one children's institution, the staff went to great effort to plan for a group of boys a long outing to view a parade. The experience was topped off with a special snack treat. The actual trip went off beautifully; the boys were on their best behavior and seemed to have fun. Back on the ward, however, the child care workers encountered glum hostility, rather than a carry-over of good spirits. The boys were cross and argumentative, both with the workers and among themselves. Like children at home, institutionalized children become depressed and quarrelsome after too much of this sort of pleasure.

As a general rule, it is better for the children to be taken ice-skating than to watch a hockey meet (except for the few real sports fans); to go Christmas caroling themselves rather than be sung to by an outside group. This type of active experience helps the children develop skills and initiative, thus increasing their self-esteem; a passive experience is more likely to reinforce their feelings of inadequacy. It is better that holiday parties be limited to the few that the children can really enjoy and that some of the community organizations that wish to give to the children at holiday times be asked to contribute in such a way as to enrich the children's daily life throughout the year—to give sports equipment for after-school use rather than tickets to a baseball game, table games and craft supplies for on-unit use rather than the third Christmas party in two days. Volunteer party givers can be surprisingly cooperative when such suggestions are tactfully made.

Visits to workers' homes constitute a special and very tricky problem. The relationship of the worker to the individual, the group, and the other workers can be jeopardized if he takes a single child to visit his home, and in general this should not be done. The one-to-one experience, perhaps pleasurable on the surface, can remind children vividly and painfully that they are away from their own families. In addition, the unverbalized hope on the part of many children that a worker may take them in permanently is unrealistically stirred up. Instead, following permission from supervisors, a group of children, rather than one, may be taken by several workers to the home of one of them. This avoids the pitfalls of the one-to-one relationship in the home visit, with the feelings and unrealistic expectations that might be aroused by it.

In one institution at Thanksgiving, most of the children went home to their families, leaving about six children who would have to stay at the institution. Two workers received permission to take these children to the home of one of them for some indoor games, cider, and doughnuts. This trip provided each child with a family-type experience away from the institution without provoking in them ungratifiable fantasies that one worker would now actually make him a member of his own family.

The child care worker who wants to give materially to an individual child does have sensible ways of doing this open to him. Sometimes workers are allowed to donate anonymously an item which they can specify for a particular child. If a worker wishes to give to the whole group, supervisors often give permission for him to bring in extra food treats for all the children. In this way the entire group has enjoyment in receiving and the worker in giving. Or he can sometimes bring in a toy or a game which is appropriate for all or most of the group; sometimes also it is suitable for him to bring a small present for every child. Before doing so, however, it is wise to check with those with an overview of the entire treatment program as to the advisability of what he proposes. Wise supervisors, understanding the desires of the workers to give and the strong need of the children to receive small individual items from their guardians, try to see that there is a supply of things like magazines, pencils, tablets, simple craft materials, etc., so that the workers can let the children have these things when the need arises.

In conclusion, many child care workers, especially at first, have a tendency to feel that they can and must make up for all the past deprivations of the youngsters by giving them gifts and developing intense personal relationships with certain ones with whom they most strongly identify. As has been pointed out, these attempts are not always in the child's best interest. But the worker can use himself to help the child grow and develop from where he is, and perhaps this is the greatest kind of giving that he can achieve. The worker who finds an envelope of Kool-Aid that has slid behind the shelf and has a group of withdrawn children mix up a batch on a hot summer evening, or the worker who discovers and retrieves a big empty carton that the children will enjoy playing with, or the one who listens and understands when the children are upset when they could be expected to be grateful, he is the worker who is truly giving to the children.

Runaways

It is a rare institution from which certain children do not attempt to run away and perhaps actually succeed in doing so. Institutions develop policies for handling the reporting of the runaway's absence, for finding him, and for handling him when he returns. The management of runaway children is often a subject that calls forth many divergent opinions among the staff members. For example, many trained child care workers have learned of the approach taken by certain smaller treatment centers where returned runaways (at least at the beginning of treatment) are welcomed back and given abundant supplies of food and such other nurturant care as they want. There is no thought of planning punitive consequences. The intent is to make the child feel that he is completely accepted by the staff and that all are happy that he is back and safe. Thus these workers may be appalled when runaways in large institutions are isolated, either in rooms or in special discipline or isolation cottages, to do nothing or to do meaningless tasks, and when they are the subject of a "how-can-we-punish-them" discussion.

This section considers a possible way of helping the worker develop an attitude that takes into account both the peculiar problem that the runaway constitutes for a large institution and also the needs of the children for hygienic handling. From a realistic point of view, the fact that in an institution there are large numbers of children to care for safely—probably with a low ratio of staff—makes it difficult to hold such a benign attitude toward children who run away or to take them back with open arms, positive as such a practice might be. In the larger setting some administrators feel that the returned runaway cannot be treated in a way that makes other children feel there are greater benefits to be gained by running away than by staying within bounds. Administrators of institutions (as well, of course, as those of smaller settings) feel a strong responsibility for the safety of the children, which is jeopardized if the children leave the area of staff supervision. In addition, administrators do not wish to be the subject of adverse publicity.

There are several ways in which an institution—and the child care worker within it—can handle a runaway in a nondestructive and hopefully growth-producing way. Most important is to consider why a child runs away, and this can always be done no matter how large the institution and no matter how many other problems are related to the incident. In many ways a child's running away can be traced to individual factors in his life situation and to his own mode of functioning. Among a group of children running away, for example, one may leave because he is worried about his family and wants to track it down; another may have been poorly accepted in the ward group and joins the "escape" in order to become "one of the boys"; another may have a poorly developed sense of reality and has simply wandered off with the others; still another may feel that his life in the institution is restricted and meaningless and is seeking more adventure.

Related to the various reasons for running away are the ways of preventing it, the ways of avoiding as much as possible the type of climate and situations which make a child want to leave. All the previously cited examples suggest means of prevention. Had the staff been sensitive to the feelings of the boy who was trying to find his family? Had the workers been able to pick up any cues from him that he was worried about them, and did they pass them on to the social workers? Had the workers been sensitive to the second child's feelings of exclusion and been devising and managing group situations so as to help him find greater acceptance? Was the child who wandered off the victim of a poor pattern of supervision so that his absence was not even noted for a while? And, finally—and this instance is most directly related to the work of the child care staff—had a consistent effort been made to inject variety, interest, and the opportunity to develop new skills into the on-unit program? This is not to say by any means that the child care worker can prevent all runaways. But the alert worker holds some elements of prevention in his grasp, even though many factors in the case of an individual child are beyond his control, resting in the wider social milieu and in the intrapsychic problems of the child.

An occasional runaway from an institution probably reflects a variety of difficulties converging in the experience of the child involved; a chronic rash of runaways and the staff's preoccupation with their management usually mean that there are unresolved tensions in the children's environment which should be investigated. For example, the element of freedom, discussed in the section of discipline, may be involved if there is a frequency of runaways. Do the children who are able to handle it have sufficient freedom to move about on their own? Conversely, for the children who need more structure in their environment are there boundaries and guidelines so that they do not wander off in confusion? Are there available spaces in the institution both for the children to be alone and for them to participate in vigorous activity?[1]

In addition to his role in preventing runaways, the child care worker frequently is involved in handling the returned child. The child care worker can use his knowledge of and his interest in the individual child to help shed light on the reasons for the child's departure by passing on useful information to supervisory and other clinical staff. It would be hoped that he would talk with the child about the reasons for his running away and help him see what everyone involved could do to improve the situation. Often the worker is responsible for the child's care on his return, helping him shower, getting him clean clothing, food, etc. Although he may not have permission or resources to offer abundant comforts, he is able to administer what he does in a benign and sympathetic way. If other staff have decided on a plan for handling the returnee that the worker does not agree with—for example, if he feels that it is too severe—while he may not be able to alter it, he can still take a warm stance toward the returning child without undermining the policies. He may say, "Gee, I'm sorry you got yourself in such a jam" or, "Things must have been making you feel pretty bad for you to want to leave like that, and I'm glad you're safe and sound." He would not say, "You should have stayed away for all the use we have for you" or, "If I had *my* way, you wouldn't have to be in the isolation room at all."

If punishment is administered, it would be hoped that it is logical and properly timed. Overlong isolation, long assignments of meaningless work, or deprivation of all activities not only increase a child's feeling of hostility toward and rejection of the institution and its staff, but also draw special attention to him as

1. The reader is referred to an example given by Eva Burmeister in her book, *Tough Times and Tender Moments in Child Care Work* (New York and London, 1967), in which a worker persuaded a child to come back to the institution after a home visit when he was prepared to overstay his leave without permission because of concern for his family.

an outcast. These factors make it even more difficult for him to resume a normal and productive course of life in the institutional program and to have positive relationships with the other children. All of this, of course, can increase his sense of hopelessness and futility and thus increase the probability that he may again leave the grounds. On the other hand, for some children it makes sense that although they will ultimately be allowed to resume their privileges, perhaps they should not be taken on the next off-grounds trip. Individualization, of course, is the prime consideration in managing the runaway. For the severely disturbed child who has just wandered off or even for the occasional nonverbal child who is a real escape artist, it is ridiculous to think in terms of isolation to teach him not to do it again.

Family Contact and Relationships

In many large institutions, the main responsibility for handling family matters is delegated to social caseworkers, who communicate and work with families. Some institutions have a set policy—and a good one, of course—that all families must be involved in ongoing casework. Other institutions, unfortunately, do not have the trained staff to offer such a service. Some institutions have blanket policies for both the child's home visits and the parents' coming to the institution, setting a certain number of allowed visits of a certain type per unit of time. Other institutions individualize visiting procedures for each child depending on the needs and circumstances of all involved. When the team approach is an integral feature of an institution's program, matters relevant to the child's contact with his family are brought up to the entire team as a part of making his treatment plan. Sometimes the psychiatrist, if there is one present, makes the decision about the child's visiting procedure, taking into account the team members' feelings, and the social worker carries out the plan developed by the team.

As a team member the child care worker offers his observations and ideas about the child's relationship with his family. As the child's "home" person in the institution, carrying out many of the functions that parents do, the worker has had the opportunity to see how the child reacts to parentlike figures, may have heard the child talk about his family, and probably has seen the child interact with his parents when they have come to visit. Perhaps he has spoken with them himself.

Thus the worker has valuable information to contribute. A warning is in order, however. The worker's impressions of the family can be colored by certain attitudes that he brings to his work. Beginning child care workers especially are highly indentified with the child and his problems: they really try to see the child's circumstances through his eyes, and they may focus so intently on the child himself that they fail to see him and his situation in a broad perspective. In addition, sometimes the worker tends to see himself as a sort of "savior," feeling that he, through his careful ministration and deep affection for the child, will save him from all the bad influences he has been under and perhaps still is; he will make the child better. In moderation, this idea may not be harmful to the worker's performance. After all, it is the worker's special feelings that make his arduous work meaningful and gratifying. But in their more intense form, these feelings can have a negative effect, particularly as they influence the worker's attitude toward the child's own family.

Thus workers often blame the child's parents—the mother in particular—and the child's "terrible homelife" for his problems, and they feel that to get better the child must be kept away totally from these bad influences. It is interesting to note the intense disagreement which arose over the case of one child among team members making plans for the children's forthcoming holiday visits. Almost all of the child care staff thought that this child should not have a visit because the home conditions were so bad—irregular meals, crowded sleeping arrangements, etc. Yet all of them were aware of the great desire that the *child* had expressed to see his family. Although of course it is sometimes true that a child has had such poor treatment at the hands of his parents that there may be little advantage in prolonged contact, most children do need and benefit from maintaining some kind of tie with their families (although many institutionalized children do not have families). It is sometimes difficult for workers who themselves were brought up with warm care in an intact family to see the merits of children's having contact with families who seem to them to have done a poor job in providing the essentials of good child-rearing. It is hard for them to see that these families still may have offered positive gratification and elements for development of the child. There is, it would seem, some truth to the "old saw" that children prefer their own families, no matter how inadequate, to the best of institutions. Perhaps the families instill a sense of belonging that an institution, by structural definition, never can.

One child who was having individual counseling sessions in an institution came from what conventionally would be called a poor home, where there was real evidence that he had been neglected and mistreated. Yet his interest in and allegiance to his family were obvious in his behavior and conversation. In his counseling sessions he was reluctant to participate in any discussion which would make it seem as if he harbored disloyal feelings. It was only when the counselor pointed out that the institution and his family were not fighting against each other but rather were both working for the same goal, his return home, that he began to open up a bit and show some of his mixed feelings about his parents.

It has been pointed out previously that children in large institutions do not always come from multiproblem families. The rejection and hostility which the workers sometimes feel they see in parents may well exist in some cases, but may exist in some of these cases as the result of years of exhausting living with a difficult child who has given little positive feedback and who may have been extremely difficult to manage. The fact that workers are not so intimately involved in their interactions with the children, are relieved periodically of responsibility for their care, and do not hold total responsibility for planning their treatment helps them to make an objective, helpful, and sympathetic approach to their charges. The children need such an attitude, of course, or they would not be in the institution, and usually they improve as they establish relationships on a new basis. But the worker should also maintain a compassionate attitude toward those people—the parents—with whom the child's relationship and ties have been so profound and who are ultimately responsible for him. If children have come from backgrounds of chronic poverty, the stresses imposed on their mother's and father's parental abilities may be difficult for middle-class workers to understand.

Those whose task it is to make clinical decisions concerning the children's family contact generally use the dimensions of quantity and quality to make plans that meet the needs and circumstances of each. Blanket policies, such as "Children may have one home visit a month" or "Parents may spend an hour with their child each Sunday," tend to make the children feel cut off from their families and the institution seem like an impersonal place, thus causing their positive adjustment to it to be more difficult. On the other hand, individualization of policy provides the staff with the opportunity to make plans which are most suitable for each child. For example, if a boy's problem has involved hostile behavior toward a baby sister and there is only one child's bedroom in the home, this child's home visits would be limited to the daytime. Or if a child gives evidence that he can hold himself together for only a certain period before "blowing up," time permitted for a visit might be very brief. If the visit is to take place on a holiday such as the Fourth of July, staff might recommend that the child be taken on a quiet country picnic rather than to the fireworks and an amusement park, thus preventing him from becoming overstimulated and ending his visit on a negative note. In each of these cases, however, the child has contact with his family of the length and kind that is best for him.

In addition to his role as a team member giving observations about the child in relationship to his family, the child care worker may have some direct contact with the child's parents. Frequently the worker is the person who meets the parents when they come to pick up the child or return him from a visit; in addition, they may exchange the child's possessions, such as finished projects, laundry, presents, food, etc. Elaboration of the dynamics inherent in some of these contacts can help the worker understand better any stress and unpleasantness he may encounter. Sometimes the worker is placed in a dilemma as the parents press him with their problems and concerns and with questions about the child's behavior.

If the parents are having a disagreement with the doctor or social worker in charge of their case, they may deliberately seek extra information and opinions from others than those through whom communication is generally channelled. It is tempting for the child care worker to want to supply his ideas, since he wants to please and is aware of his special knowledge. From the point of view of treatment, however, the policy in most institutions is for the worker to redirect the parent to those directly concerned with parent work. If the worker is asked, for example, "Do you think Johnny is getting anything out of his school program?" almost always the answer is something like, "I suggest that you talk to his social worker, who has the teacher's latest reports"; or if the worker is asked, "Do you think that scratch on Jimmy's knee was treated properly?" again the most appropriate response is something like, "The doctor or the nurse could discuss this with you."

The worker should understand that such a policy of his not giving direct information is not the result of any feeling that he is incapable of handling the situation; rather, allowing the parent to seek various opinions dilutes and undermines his relationship with the caseworker and contributes toward the type of confused communication and misunderstanding that can so easily develop and is not therapeutic to anyone. The worker should always be sympathetic, however, when parents complain of the care their child is receiving, even if he, the worker, seems to be the object of their complaint. He should not take the parents' complaint personally, nor become involved in their feelings (if he does so, he may risk turning his own feelings on the child). Always the worker should refer the complaint to the proper person—the director of the unit, the doctor, or the social worker. Often workers do receive permission to answer parents' questions about the children's interests on the unit, for example, "Jane really enjoys the dolls you sent her a few weeks ago" or "Tim swam in the deep water for the first time last week," but even before going this far, the worker should check with supervisors first.

While some parents may be very friendly to the worker, others may be inexplicably hostile, seeming to find fault with anything they can—the child's grooming, state of nourishment, mood, etc. Here again there is often an explanation. If the child seems to be developing positive relationships with the staff and making progress in the program, the parents often have mixed feelings. On the one hand, of course, they are happy that their child is improving. On the other, it is not easy for parents to see their child making progress in the care of strangers that he was not able to make when they, the parents, were caring for him. Workers, especially if they are parents themselves, can often put themselves in the place of the parents and understand something of what they are feeling.

Much worker-child interaction goes on around the visits of the parents. The worker prepares the child emotionally and physically for the visit; the child may be feeling either anticipation or anxiety, and often a combination of both. He perhaps understands that he is living at the institution because his behavior has been of a kind that could not be easily managed at home. If his behavior has improved, he may wonder if his parents will take him home to live soon. If it has not, he may fear that they will never come again. These thoughts may not be articulated in the child's mind, but he may show that something is bothering him. (The reader is referred to the example of Bobby in the section "Response to Feelings" in chapter 3.) After the visit the worker helps the child to work out his feelings—homesickness, the renewed loss of his parents, disappointment. As they talk, worker and child in a sense assess the visit. It may have been a happy one, or relatively so. It may truly have been an unhappy one, but if the child reports that it was unhappy, the worker needs to consider this report in the light of the youngster's own attitudes—

his need for the worker's indulgence, his need perhaps to retaliate against his parents. If the worker finds his indignation rising at the child's account of what was said and done during the visit, he should take his own feelings with a grain of salt. After all, this is a one-sided account.

Sex Behavior and Interests

Sex concerns arise in the lives of all children, whether they live at home, in boarding schools or camps, in one of the shelters for victims of family disruption, or in another sort of institution. School-age children are naturally secretive about their sex interests, and in ordinary circumstances much of their sex talk and behavior is concealed from adults. When children live in an institution under the constant supervision of child care workers, their natural sex behavior and curiosity are exposed, and the adults must respond to it because they are adults and because they have both a child-care and a legal commitment to the welfare of the children. The past circumstances of institutionalized children's lives have in some cases heightened their interest in sexual matters, but their developmental gaps and lack of contact with the neighborhood group have often left them more ignorant than other children. Thus the worker may encounter expressions, questions, and behavior which not only shock him or at least catch him off guard but often require some kind of action.

The worker should avoid regarding the sex behavior he sees in terms of morality. It is not a question of whether the behavior or the child is good or bad. Rather, the concern is to try to understand the meaning of the child's behavior and to handle it in such a way as to promote his healthy growth. This does not, it should be emphasized, mean that the behavior should always be permitted; often it should not. It does mean that the worker has to be aware of the meanings of the behavior in an institutional group setting and of ways, if necessary, to prevent, rechannel, and/or discuss it with the children that are appropriate to the situation and to the individuals in it.

Masturbation and exploratory activity or sex play are the commonest types of sexual behavior encountered in the institution. The worker need not interfere immediately with masturbation unless the child is doing it in public. In the residence, however, the worker may want to redirect the youngster's activity if it makes him the object of ridicule or abuse by the other children. The child who masturbates constantly or in such a way that he seems to be experiencing pain rather than pleasure may be expressing an unusual degree of anxiety. If he has individual therapy, help can perhaps come from that source; but in any case the workers should try to consider if anything in the child's institutional life might make him feel under pressure. And, as will be suggested below, they should see that he has other things to do; children sometimes masturbate simply out of boredom. (Children who have nothing to do sometimes also pick at sores, press their bruises, play with saliva, and so on.) Sometimes children masturbate because it is the only way they know of giving themselves pleasure, and it is often possible to help them find other pleasurable activities. Finally, a child occasionally goes off by himself to masturbate as a means of "pulling himself together," and if this seems to be the case, the worker should not interfere.

Often institutionalized children who initiate sexual contact with each other are actually seeking physical closeness to another human being. These may be children who have had little mothering in their past lives but who may have had premature exposure to adult sexual activity, either through observing adults or through having adults make advances to them. Thus they translate their need for close human contact into sexual terms, since this may have been the only form in which they have experienced it in the past. When two children are discovered together in sex play, it is usually best that they be separated, but this can be done in a matter-of-fact manner without scolding or shaming. It is especially urgent for the workers to see that no child is exploited against his will and that a younger child is not taken advantage of by an older one even with his consent. When contacts are made between children of the same sex, the worker does need to bear in mind that these incidents do not mean that the children involved will grow up to be homosexuals. Such episodes sometimes occur in the everyday life of the school-age child; they are a feature of his developmental level.

It is sensible for the workers to encourage the kind of unit climate which provides wholesome activity appropriate for the age level and does not deliberately provide situations which encourage sex play. In this endeavor, programming is very important. Children with too little exercise and too little opportunity for enjoyable play or children allowed to spend too much time drifting around or sitting in a solitary corner are the ones most likely to be preoccupied with sex activity. Children growing up in a normal setting drain off much of their energy—including their "sex" energy—in active play: wrestling, running games, swimming, organized sports. Some of these things can be provided in the institution; workers can structure supervised wrestling, tag, tumbling, pillow fights, water play, wagon-pushing, jungle-gym climbing, as well as catch, basket-throwing, and more organized games according to the children's ability.

Grouping of the children is also important. For example, one would not place a boy known to be sexually aggressive in the same sleeping room with a passive, fearful boy who would not be able to defend himself or protest against unwelcome approaches. Two children who excite each other by colorful language might be placed at different tables in the dining room. In handling toileting, bathing, and preparation for bedtime, the workers should provide for privacy for those who want it and should, as much as possible, avoid insisting that children of different stages of physical development expose themselves to one another. Such circumstances can sometimes be too stimulating for some of those involved.

An often-overlooked aspect of dealing with sexual behavior in children is the role of some workers in unconsciously encouraging it. Uniforms for child care workers are discussed more fully in another section, but it can be mentioned here, for example, that they can be truly helpful in preventing young female workers from being seen as sex objects by preadolescent and adolescent boys and in being able to establish a professional relationship with them.

Frequently one encounters in institutions little girls who have learned before being institutionalized to employ seductive mannerisms to make their way in the world. It is easy for uninitiated male workers to respond in kind to their flirtatious approaches, which may be totally inappropriate for their age. These little girls need to have male workers available to them who can help them learn appropriate ways of behaving toward men by responding warmly but not in a way that mirrors the child's flirtatious behavior.

Finally, in their wish to give to the children, workers may gratify their requests for some kind of clothing or freedom that is unsuitable at their stage of development.

A little girl was just beginning to learn new and more appropriate ways of interacting with boys and men, which were in contrast to her behavior at the time she came in. She had begun to notice the physical development of the older girls who were beginning to wear brassieres. She asked the women workers for one, although she was only nine years old with corresponding lack of physical development. The workers brought her one on the sly. The supervisor needed to talk to the workers about how they were only encouraging the type of older behavior that everybody had been working to discourage. She suggested that they take an approach with the child that showed her that she was highly regarded and acceptable as a girl of her age and that when her body had matured like that of the older girls, she too would be able to wear the same kind of clothing they did.

Workers will undoubtedly be asked questions and encounter situations which show that the children have a real need for proper sex instruction and explanation. In the large setting, where the children may be having numerous contacts with people of whom they can ask questions, it is often wise for the workers to consult their supervisors and unit team before going into extensive explanations. It is important that the approach taken in educating the children be a consistent one and that all staff are more or less agreed on what information is given and how it is presented. Otherwise the children will invade with questions those people who they perceive will give different answers and thus often increase their own confusion. If the worker feels from things that have been happening in the group that the children either lack information or have misinformation, he can do a great service by informing the supervisor and the team of his suspicions so that an appropriate educational program can be instituted. Many institutions expend considerable energy in preventing or suppressing any expression of interest in sexual matters when they might more effectively offer an educational program which can suitably explain and deal with the concerns that the children show.

Although a child should receive a straightforward answer appropriate to his stage of development as soon as possible after asking a question, it is not always "begging the question" in an institutional setting for the worker to tell the child that he will discuss the matter at another time—naming the time if at all possible. This gives the worker time to check what the best way of handling the question might be for the particular child. The worker's decision on how to handle the individual question will be partially based on his perception of what is going on in the entire group at the time it is posed. A question asked while the group is having a quiet bedtime snack will be dealt with differently from one that is shouted across the dining room.

One child was extremely interested in the pregnancy of the unit supervisor, with whom she had a stormy but meaningful relationship. She had a legitimate need for information, and the supervisor often talked to her individually, but when both were with the group, the child often used her interest to stir up the rest of the group to hilarity by asking personal questions with poorly smothered giggles. At these times the supervisor simply told her she would talk privately with her later. When they were alone, the child was able to attend appropriately, and they had many meaningful discussions.

A discussion with a whole group whose sex concerns are similar may be equally fruitful.

A new young male worker was in charge of a group of verbal school-age boys as they played with clay. He was the first new male worker to be employed since the boys had been admitted, and, as always happens, the group began to test him. They all were rolling the clay to look like snakes. One of the youngsters held up his snake and called it by one of the slang words for penis. Another boy then fashioned his roll to make it look more like an actual penis. The new worker, concerned as to how he should handle this, became quite anxious—as the boys undoubtedly perceived. They continued to test, teasing him by holding up their long rolls and calling them a pencil, a rod, a rifle. Finally the worker said, "Okay, so you're all talking about a penis. We all have one." There were gales of rather embarrassed laughter from the boys. One of them jumped up and danced around holding the clay in front of his pants. Finally the worker confronted the situation and said, "Quit dancing around and come over here and talk." When all were sitting at the table, he said, "We don't have very much time now, because we have to clean up this clay and get ready for supper, but if you boys really want to talk about this, I'll try to see that you get a chance."

Since he worked in a large institution, with many people involved in the children's treatment, he mentioned this incident to his supervisor when he went off duty and was encouraged to go ahead with the subject, since the boys had obviously turned to him with their concerns. When he gathered them around the table the next day, there was at first much hilarity. He was assaulted by personal questions: Did he have a girl friend? Did he ever take her to bed with him? These he handled as well as he could by saying that his personal affairs were his own business and he was not going to talk about them, but if they had other questions, he would be glad to discuss them. Gradually the giggling began to subside and a couple of the boys began to reveal assaultive fantasies about the sex act. You would have to beat a woman, they supposed, to get her to have sex with you. The worker said that women can enjoy sex too, that two people have to know each other very well, and then if they both want to have sex, both can enjoy it. This conversation led to several others, all initiated by the boys. The worker occasionally found himself in perplexity and would sometimes ask advice of old hands on the staff, but mainly he was guided by his own good sense.

The question of what type of boy-girl relationships are appropriate inevitably crops up in an institutional setting. How much supervision should boys and girls have? What kind of relationships and activities should be permitted or encouraged? This is a complicated topic which cannot be completely covered here, although a few general matters can be discussed. It would certainly seem appropriate that the boys and girls have contact with one another in school and recreation, much as they do in the larger community. How much unstructured time boys and girls share and how the time is used are usually dependent on two things, the philosophy of the administration and the characteristics and degree of disturbance of the group.

Although almost all administrators of modern institutions would probably agree that total segregation is unrealistic and does not serve to promote healthy development, there are some who do feel that contacts should be carefully planned and supervised. Most administrators would not allow adolescents to drift into situations in which intimate contact could take place; however, they would support arrangements in which boys and girls can be together where there is general supervision but where the adolescents need not have the feeling that they are being eavesdropped upon. One institution initiated a conversation hour, when the adolescent boys and girls could get together informally, with adults at a distance, to talk to one another and to share refreshments. In those (usually small) treatment centers where staff patterns and semiautonomous groups allow family style living, boys and girls can share living quarters, and it is the responsibility of the workers to see that the relations between them do not go beyond what would be acceptable in a family. But just as the style of living in a large institution differs widely from that in a family, so must the rules governing the relationship between boys and girls. The living arrangements must take into account the youngsters whose behavior may be extreme, as well as those of more moderate habits. Thus older boys and girls, at least in large institutions, have separate living quarters, and the staff must make a conscious effort to provide boy-girl contacts. Because, unless there is careful planning, there may be many more opportunities in some institutions for youngsters to get into trouble than there is in the community, the workers are concerned to provide the opportunity for acceptable behavior, to reinforce it when it occurs, and to redirect behavior which is not acceptable.

Caring for Other Children

Brief mention was made in chapter 7 of the practice of having some children in the institutional living unit help with the care of others who are younger or more inadequate. There are certain aspects to this practice which warrant careful consideration. Sometimes older children receive gratification out of participating in the care of younger ones whom they can mother and give to. This type of relationship can have real benefits both to the children and to the staff, but only if it is allowed under carefully controlled circumstances and under careful supervision. Under proper conditions, the need to feel important, useful, and close to others can be met for the older children and extra contact and stimulation provided for the younger ones. But when the arrangement is made haphazardly, the results can be untherapeutic and even tragic.

First, even though some older children may maintain that they are interested in helping to care for the smaller ones, or the staff feels that this would be a constructive experience, too much dependence on the older children makes inroads on their time, which they should perhaps be spending on appropriate age-level activities. In addition, often having been deprived of close contact in the past, they can give just so much to others before they have "had their fill" themselves. If these children are left unsupervised with younger children or made to be with them for too long, their own feelings of anger and deprivation come to the surface and are then translated into aggressive and bullying behavior toward their charges. This behavior is in contrast to the real gentleness and concern which they can show when this kind of experience is carefully planned and structured for them. It is poor judgment to have older children without supervision bathe and dress younger ones, since this situation can be overstimulating to all involved, none of whom may have the knowledge or the ego-strength to manage appropriately.

The older children often function best in helping younger ones in activities or semiacademic work, which allow them to show their skills and knowledge. Girls sometimes enjoy helping to feed and escort younger children, hugging them and holding their hands in the process. If done under supervision and in such a way that the younger children's need to grow and explore is not intruded upon, this help is often reasonable to allow.

One quite withdrawn small boy lived on a unit in which there were also several preadolescent girls. In great need of stimulation in order to develop, he received much help through the interest taken in him by these girls. Sometimes they would mother him, appealing to his need for warmth, but at other just as important times they would encourage him to do something and express their pleasure if he did: "Hey, Jean [the worker], do you know what Ronnie just did? He put the truck puzzle together all by himself!" The positive attitudes of the girls toward this child were helpful to all involved—the girls themselves, the boy, and the workers, whose interest in Ronnie was engaged further by what the girls helped him to do.

Pets

It is sometimes proposed that a unit pet be obtained for institutionalized children as a way to help meet their need for contact and to give them a neutral object upon which to lavish affection and care. As in the matter of the older children's helping the younger ones, this can be either a therapeutic success or a tragic disaster, depending on how it is handled. Workers often request a pet for the unit; before doing so and before making a commitment to it, they should be aware of the broader implications of having a pet in a children's institution.

Adults introducing a pet into a children's living area (often in the large institution medical clearance must be obtained first) must have an established plan by which they can be responsible for providing twenty-four-hour-a-day, seven-day-a-week care and protection to the animal, including ample space both for exercise and for withdrawal from the attentions of the children. In other words, the child care workers must be prepared to assume the responsibility for the care of the pet as well as of the children, since disturbed children, even more than normal ones, at times lose interest and thus become unpredictable in offering consistent care to the pet.

The animal should be a sturdy one, well able to get away from active, possibly aggressive children and to withstand vigorous treatment without becoming retaliatory. The usual tiny kitten is a poor choice in most situations. From the pet's point of view, it is not fair to subject it to abuse. From the point of view of the children, their unresolved feelings of anger are often taken out on a helpless animal; if an animal actually is killed or severely injured by the children, unfortunate consequences result. The child who is responsible may gain further evidence for any fantasies he may have regarding his ability to be totally destructive (many disturbed children have such fantasies). Besides, the rest of the group is angry, and the children's relationships suffer.

If, however, the workers are able to provide the pattern of supervision and the kind of pet that would preclude the possibility of the children's injuring or abusing it and if the children are ready to have a pet—if they have sufficient control and orientation to cope with an animal living with them—then the pet can be a positive force in their development. For children too shy or withdrawn to relate to other children or to grown-ups, the pet offers a wonderful recipient for their first advances. The care of, and antics of, the pet provide an excellent means of drawing staff and children together as they plan for its care and watch its playful activity. The pet provides an additional dimension to the children's lives and certainly can counteract the tendency for a unit to appear cold and institutional. Presence of an animal *under proper circumstances* can bring out feelings of concern, sympathy, and empathy in the children who in the past have had little opportunity to develop or express these sentiments.

Uniforms

In some institutions, particularly hospital settings, the child care workers are required to wear uniforms; in others they are not. Whatever the practice may be in the institution where he is, the worker will want to understand some of the thinking behind the decision. Of late years many administrators of children's units have come to feel that uniforms make their workers look too official, and they expect them instead to appear in neat, informal washable attire. The reasoning behind this change is that a more homelike atmosphere is maintained when the workers wear ordinary dress and, too, that the white hospitallike uniform is unsuitable for workers who may perhaps sit on the floor or the grass with the children, may be helping the children use clay or finger paint, and may often hold a dirty and upset child in their arms. Skirts and blouses for the women and slacks and sport shirts for the men are more functional because they show the dirt less and because the worker need not always be protecting the whiteness of his costume.

There are, however, some arguments in favor of the uniform. Some administrators feel that for children who are confused and poorly oriented—and this is, of course, characteristic of many disturbed institutionalized children—the uniform helps them to identify the workers' function and thus to sort out their environment better. In large institutions where there are so many different people to whom the child is exposed, this idea is particularly applicable. If workers are close in age to the children being treated (college students working with older adolescents, for example), the uniforms are helpful to the workers and to the children in differentiating the two groups and in making the authority of the worker more meaningful. The younger worker can perhaps best see himself in a worker image when he is wearing a uniform; for the young female worker assigned to preadolescent and adolescent boys, the standardized and somewhat more sedate appearance provided by a uniform can serve a similar purpose and keep the boys from seeing her as a peer whom it is appropriate to approach flirtatiously. (The administrator who believes in the "no-uniform" practice would expect the workers to establish their role by their attitudes toward the children, rather than their dress.)

In some institutions, compromises have been worked out. Some administrators find it feasible for workers to wear uniforms for most daily duties but to have considerable freedom to change to civilian clothing when they accompany children on various activities. In other places women workers may wear a colorful standardized uniform which is not hospital white but which differentiates them from the children.

It would seem as if there are a variety of factors to be weighed by the workers as they consider their feelings about uniforms. As in so many aspects of child development and child care, there is no set way of looking at the situation.

CHAPTER 10

The Worker and Institutional Policies: Property and Records

Property

The handling of property—both the child's and the institution's—is a prime function of the child care worker and one frequently governed by institutional policies. The following section covers several aspects of this dimension of child care in an institution.

Care and cleanup. Chapter 4 emphasizes the importance of caring for the children's possessions and play materials and of keeping them intact. The worker who snatches from a shelf a game with pieces missing (as a result of poor supervision of an earlier play session) and slams it on a table for the children to get themselves started and figure out what to do can expect to reap chaos and destruction. The one who sits down with an intact set of materials and begins to involve the children stands a better chance of promoting a pleasant, constructive time; and having lent himself to the children's activity for a period, he may then be able to move away to something else if necessary. A part of the responsibility for cleanup and housekeeping belongs to the child care worker. In most institutions the workers, with the help of the children, put away toys and activity materials and in this process can make sure that no parts of games or other small objects are lost among the trash. Cleaning up after activities involves throwing away wastepaper and other trash and mopping up paint that has dripped, and with these activities also the children can help.

In a large institution the responsibility for heavy housekeeping duties is usually that of a separate janitorial or housekeeping department. Sometimes a difficult situation is created between the child care staff and the housekeeping staff, who may feel that the workers allow the children to be too messy, thus making additional work for them. The workers should be aware that housekeepers, maids, and janitors derive their sense of accomplishment from doing their job well—keeping things neat and orderly—just as the workers derive satisfaction from seeing the children get better. Ultimately, of course, the needs of the children come first, and for clinical reasons sometimes supervisors need to clarify goals and work out solutions for reaching objectives. But the on-the-spot worker also has a role in attempting to prevent such conflicts from arising. He must try to see objectively if there might really be some justification for the complaints. Was sloppy or destructive activity permitted to the point where it really was not beneficial to the children or where it was really damaging to property? No activity should be undertaken that will result in a "mess" that is beyond the power of the workers to clean up.

Some workers feel that a general air of disorder, characterized by lost, broken, and scattered toys and other materials and ripped and marked walls, denote a "free" environment where children can be creative. This is not really the case. Such disorganization in the physical surroundings usually contributes to disorganization in thinking and behavior. Workers do need to help the children maintain in the living area what one might call "comfortable order"—a sufficient lack of rigidity so that the children can enjoy their activities, yet not so much lack of care and control that property is destroyed as the result of chaotic behavior toward it.

The workers can also help in their day-to-day contacts with the housekeeping and janitorial staff by engaging this group's interests in the ongoing progress of the children whom they see and with whom they have at least indirect contact.

The housekeeping staff in an institution were annoyed one day when they noticed a puddle of urine on their newly cleaned floor. The worker explained (as he cleaned up the puddle) how this accident indirectly represented progress on the part of the child involved. He had been wearing diapers, which had avoided evidence of his not being trained, but the workers had felt he was ready to advance to training pants. This was the first slip back, when he did not make it to the bathroom on time. When this was explained to the housekeepers, their annoyance diminished and instead they developed an interest in the progress of this particular child.

Safety restrictions. The area that contains medications and records, the nursing station in hospital units, is, of course, off limits to the children. Unfortunately this area is often the gathering place where child care staff and others communicate and do unit chores, and is where the workers often sit to write their daily reports. The workers are sometimes distressed because while they are there, the children often signal their need for either material or psychological assistance; yet to have the children join them in this office or station is legitimately against policy since the dangerous substances and confidential records are exposed. The rules must be kept in mind. At least one worker should be with the children while the other or others are writing reports or doing other necessary chores. If one of the workers in the nursing station sees that a child is in need of him, he must leave the station and go to the child, not bring the child into the nursing station.

Activity materials which might be dangerous to the children if used without supervision must be kept in a locked closet or storeroom. Such things include scissors, objects made of glass, very heavy objects, and glues and cosmetics containing chemicals. Sometimes certain items of clothing such as stockings and belts are not permitted without supervision. Toys and equipment that contain dangerous parts are forbidden. It may seem to the worker that there is sometimes too much administrative rigidity about the safety policy. Yet when there is a large group of seriously disturbed children, the problem of protecting them from danger is a real one. If the pattern of supervision is spotty, if the children are going through an upset period, and if the group is large, it is sensible for the workers to be especially alert about what the children have access to.

Although the safety of the children through the storage of

materials and area restriction is important, it need not be accomplished at the expense of drab, institutional surroundings. It is possible with thought and effort to maintain both a rich and a safe environment. The child care worker who can combine the two for his group is the one who can make a *real* contribution to positive development. He can familiarize himself with all possible play materials that are safe and try to see that they are available. He can make an effort to organize his time and activities so that he is able to supervise carefully anything that is not totally safe, so that the children do not miss out completely on exposure to these materials. His attitude of caring about making materials available will carry over to the children and hopefully even to other staff. Members of different shifts of workers must communicate with one another and work out a reasonably consistent policy as to what is considered dangerous and what is not.

While on a picnic off the grounds, members of the day shift in one institution did not supervise certain aspects of the activity closely, because they thought the children should be "trusted completely." A few hours after the group's return, members of the evening shift received an excited phone call from the activities department, which had lent the picnic equipment. When the returned equipment was checked, two sharp-pronged roasting forks were discovered to be missing, and it was felt that perhaps the children had taken them. It was necessary for the evening shift to assume the unpleasant and unfortunate duty of searching both the unit and the individual children to try to find the missing forks. This was ultimately more of a setback in developing the children's trust than would have been careful supervision of the forks and checking on them before the group's return to the institution. In addition, the evening-shift workers were justifiably resentful of being put in the position where they had to search the youngsters. It turned out in the end that the forks were not on the unit but had been hidden at the picnic area by two of the boys.

Incidentally, if a search of this sort really must be undertaken, unless the object that is missing is really dangerous, each child's room should be searched in his presence. This procedure will at least minimize the loss of trust between worker and child;

it means that the worker is concerned and that the child is respected. (Do not assume, however, that the child will just sit there quietly while you search.)

It would seem most appropriate for access to areas and equipment to depend on the quality and quantity of staff coverage and on the overall mood and interest of the children. At times of minimal coverage, one may have to sacrifice certain kinds of programming for safety's sake, whereas things can be more relaxed at other times. Workers should be aware not only of what is safe, but also of the fact that different types of materials evoke different kinds of behavior from the children. Using these considerations as a basis for programming is truly good child care work. For example, clay often leads disturbed children into regressed behavior which may not be desired at a certain time; therefore, a more structured activity might be offered, such as blocks or puzzles. A small, hard ball presented to children in a confined space is likely soon to lead to an unsafe situation and the necessity for restriction, while a plastic ball, wiffle ball, or frisbee could be played with safely and freely.

Keys. An ubiquitous feature of institutional life is keys, which are needed for access but are symbols of restraint and confinement. The new worker in the institution may be amazed—and uneasy—when he goes on duty to receive a jangling ring of keys to elevators, cupboards, floors, and buildings. He may feel like a jailer as he makes his way to his place of duty, locking and unlocking doors as he goes. The feelings aroused in some workers by the possession of keys are often shared by the children, some of whom, the worker soon finds, are preoccupied with these keys, which may be to them strong symbols of feared adult authority or of containment. Children often ask workers to be allowed to hold or carry their keys and to open the door, and the workers, feeling awkward and guilty in their position of having keys, sometimes try to appease their feelings by letting the children have them either briefly or for a longer period of time. Almost always the prevailing institutional policy is for the children never to handle keys. In addition to the psychological consequences, real dangers are involved. Workers have been known to be locked in rooms by children who were then free to roam at will. Besides, permission to handle keys is not the best recognition of growth and development in individual children.

What can the worker do to handle the children's behavior and interest centered around keys? First of all, he can be honest with the children. He can acknowledge that he understands how it bothers them always to be behind locked doors and to have access to certain areas only by means of the worker-held keys. He can also explain to them that there are reasons, which have to do with their own safety and protection, for their not having the keys. There is no reason why a child cannot have a functioning key and lock, for instance on a chest which holds his own toys, and younger children can often enjoy their own set of plastic keys on a chain.

Stealing and destruction. Stealing and destruction are issues in institutional life with which the child care workers frequently must deal. Stealing occurs often in institutional settings and is brought to light when somebody reports missing property. This situation is almost always difficult to handle so that property can be safely restored but children are not humiliated by false accusations.

Prevention is the first step. The workers can protect, by keeping in a special place, anything they or the children feel might be tempting to others. Workers' pocketbooks must be locked up. The worker may contribute his suggestion to supervisory staff that each child should have his own storage space, perhaps with a lock. Of course, as has been said so many times, the best prevention is to try to see, through the programming for everyday life, that the children have their needs for interesting activities fulfilled and that they have access to an adequate amount of play material so that they have a sense of possession of these things. But taking things is so frequently symptomatic of disturbed children that it is not always possible to prevent its occurring.

If a worker suspects that something has been stolen, his first step should not be to search the unit and the children's belong-

ings while they are not there—unless, of course, the missing item
is something dangerous, in which case he must conduct a search
immediately; the children will understand the necessity for this.
If the workers choose as a first resort to ask the children about
the missing items, it is best to ask *every* child *privately*. If just a
few are asked, they feel as if they are being singled out, and their
feelings toward adults, as well as their status with the group, are
not improved. It is even more of a mistake to ask a few children
in front of the entire group. Even if they admit their guilt, it is an
unnecessarily humiliating experience. The same thinking applies
to asking all the children as a group who is guilty. In many cases
the group code is so strong that, to protect one another, they all
refuse to admit anything, or else the scapegoats in the group
are accused, rightly or wrongly. If the worker makes such grim
threats as "Nobody is going to leave this room until I know who
took the candy," he may finally exact a confession but only at the
price of losing the respect of the children and humiliating those
who confess. The children as a group can be told, however, that
if they want to talk to the worker about the missing item, he will
be happy to listen in private.

When the worker is aware that a certain child has something
that does not belong to him, he can take him aside for a life-space
interview, and this situation is ideal for this kind of interview to
be effective.

One child who had a problem of taking things began to display anything he had stolen rather conspicuously in the living area as if he
wanted the workers to notice and help him with his problem. One
time he brought in a large sheaf of paper just like that used in the
school. When the worker said gently that it looked just like the kind
of paper they had in school, the child readily said that he had taken
it while the teacher wasn't looking. The worker suggested that the
child return the paper to the schoolroom and offered to go along and
wait outside the door while the child replaced it. If the teacher was
there, the child could say that he had taken the paper but now felt
that he should put it back. The worker assured the child that the
teacher would understand.

The worker can thus help the child who steals by showing him that his problem is recognized and that the staff want to help him with it. He can enable the child to recognize the possible consequences of his actions and provide an opportunity for restitution in a way that does not degrade or humiliate him.

Destruction is another frequent occurrence in institutional life which the worker must often deal with directly. Chapters 7 and 8 describe the many ways of preventing the kind of climate which promotes destructive behavior. When overt destruction of institutional property has occurred (not through the neglect of the staff), it is often sensible for the child to make restitution if he can. The restitution should be reasonable in terms of what the child is capable of doing, without having him miss out in areas of important needs. Such a plan assumes also that the child is at a stage of development where restitution is meaningful to him. For example, if a group of children write on the walls, it is reasonable for workers to have them clean the walls, during a time when they would normally be on the living unit.

When a child destroys something belonging to another child, a more difficult situation is created. The worker should try to see what made this happen and how it could have been prevented; the circumstances under which the destruction occurred are particularly important. The angry worker is sometimes tempted to make the guilty child give one of his favorite possessions to the other child. This is usually not good practice, since it does not help the offending child learn to feel more favorable toward others. Sometimes there is a good chance for the worker to have a life-space interview with the child, indicating to him the seriousness of the situation: "Johnny is pretty unhappy that you broke the truck that he liked so much" and perhaps, "What do you think you can do to make it up to him?" The worker must be sure the child does not want to make too much restitution—such as dumping the contents of his own toy chest at Johnny's feet—as sometimes a disturbed child is wont to do. Sometimes through a discussion with both children, the worker can help them work out a satisfactory solution.

When a child consistently destroys his own property, or tries to do so, his behavior is probably related to the kinds of feelings he has about himself. If the child is in counseling, his therapist may be able to suggest ways in which the worker can help the child to manage himself. In any case a reasonable procedure is to try to prevent the child from self-destructive acts and to say, "I like what you have [or have made] and want to help you protect it." If the child really seems to need something upon which to vent angry feelings, the worker perhaps can offer a substitute. "I don't want you to rip up your new book, but here's an old magazine if you feel like tearing something." A child who destroys his own things has an extremely poor self-concept; any relationship or activity which helps him feel like an achieving and accepted person helps to deter this symptomatic behavior.

Clothing

Children's clothing involves the ownership of both the institution and the children themselves. It is a subject that is often not assigned the importance it deserves in therapeutic institutional care. Children are aware of their appearance and of the image that it transmits to the world. Some children bring their own clothing to the institution, where it becomes the institution's responsibility to care for it. Frequently difficulties arise, for the child, or the child's family, may feel that the clothing is not well cared for by the laundry and that the child's choice of wearing apparel is restricted. Other children receive "state" clothing if they are not supplied through their family or social agency. These children may resent not having their own clothing to wear, especially if their dress is inappropriate in style, is drab, and lacks variety.

Although there are some aspects of the children's clothing over which the worker has little or no control, there are others which come more directly under his jurisdiction. For one thing, there is a general appearance in clothing that makes children feel comfortable and yet appropriately dressed. This is usually a compromise between an ultra neat and clean uniform type of clothing and totally dishevelled, poorly fitting clothing. The worker can help the child achieve this happy medium through his attitudes and his practices. Both extremes communicate to the child what his guardians feel about him. Poorly cared for clothing and extremely poor efforts at grooming convey to a child that he is not cared for much; an overemphasis on neatness and orderliness makes him feel that appearances are more important than his welfare. For example, a half-tucked-in shirt is almost considered symbolic of the typical active boy. If the interaction between the workers and a boy is a constant reminder to "tuck in your shirt," then standards are too rigid; if the shirt is too small, has no buttons, and is faded and indifferently laundered, the importance of clothing to the child's self-concept has been grossly underestimated. No matter what the quality and quantity of clothing provided, the worker can take an interest in the children's overall grooming and help them make the best of what they have. The worker can help the more withdrawn children tie their shoes so that they look better and can get around better. He (or perhaps rather she) can grab a needle and thread and tack on the button that is just about to drop off a shirt. As a child is rushing by, he can pull out and arrange the collar that was crumpled inside a shirt.

The worker can give the child whenever possible the opportunity to choose what he will wear. At times the worker may have to structure appropriate choices. For example, some girls may want to wear slacks to school when the rule is for skirts or dresses. The worker has to say no to slacks but can give the girls a choice of several dresses. If workers are accustomed to selecting and laying out the children's clothing for the next day the night before, perhaps they can try to initiate a practice of having the children participate in this selection. The worker may have to tolerate some fads in the children's clothing preferences, such as wearing buttons, different color shoelaces, etc. Particularly if the clothing the children have available is of a standard, uniform type, the workers can try to accept within reasonable limits the children's attempts to put an individual touch on it. In fact, the worker can encourage the making of special touches for the children's clothing, either on or off the unit. Children can make small items of wearing apparel, such as purses, comb cases, wallets, necklaces, pins, bracelets, beanies, etc. Sometimes a cooperative occupational therapy department will furnish the unit with materials for these things or it will help the children make them if the workers let their needs be known.

Older children especially can help with the care of their clothing, and this involvement often helps them invest interest in their own appearance. In one institution the quality of the grooming of a group of adolescent girls, as well as their morale, improved remarkably when, as a result of persistent efforts from the child care staff, the girls were allowed to wash some of their own clothes instead of having them sent to the laundry, which did not always treat delicate items in the way the girls would have liked. An iron and board were secured for their use under supervision.

Finally, the worker can keep track of the status of each child's clothing and, using whatever channels are available, keep the administrative staff informed of his clothing needs. The child care worker, more than anyone, is able to see the meaning that clothing has for each individual child and to make attempts to have the children's clothing needs fulfilled.

Case Records

Child care workers in large institutions are by policy sometimes not allowed access to the children's permanent files; other institutions permit them to look at these records. When the workers are forbidden to read the children's case folders, they sometimes have negative feelings; they resent this indication of low status and feel that it prevents them from having information which they should have in order to provide the best care for the children. It is easy to sympathize with the workers' feeling that they do not "rate" access to the records. If they are expected to contribute their reports and observations to the case file, they should, it would seem, be able to share the other information in it, especially since they are the people who spend the greatest amount of time with the children.

Divorcing the issue of access to the records from the problem of the status of the workers, however, it is appropriate to discuss how much information the worker needs to work effectively with the children. Optimally, the worker should know something about the child's background, his family relationships, the kind of problems he had before he came to the institution, what his personality and intellectual characteristics are, his basic health history, and particularly the goals of treatment and the treatment plan. In all honesty the worker may not need to know everything about the child in great detail in order to respond appropriately and therapeutically to him. If the worker is given a general description of the child's personality structure and level of intellectual functioning, for example, it may not be necessary for him to see all the psychological test protocols from which these descriptions were derived. The child care worker must, however, receive at least the type of information described above in order to do an adequate job, from whatever source it can be provided, case records or other.

Administrators in one institution answered the justified request of unit child care workers for more background information on their children by supplying abstracts from their psychosocial history, psychological test report, and treatment recommendations from the intake evaluation conference. These summaries of a sheet or two were placed on the unit in each child's ward folder. Thus all workers could have access to the most important and relevant information whenever they needed it.

This chapter and the two preceding ones have examined in some detail certain representative aspects of institutional life. These are areas in which institutions must develop guiding policies and procedures; they are areas in which child care workers must operate in their everyday work with the children. The reader may feel after such an extensive briefing on institutional procedures that life in an institution is simply a network of policies to be applied. Rather, where there are large groups of children and a large number of diverse adults involved in providing their total care, these inevitable policies are simply guidelines for working in such a way that everyone's function is supportive of the total effort. During one's day-to-day life in caring for institutionalized children, the activity, the change, and the variety in contact with other people provide the context against which the child care worker does his job. An understanding of the function of the procedures around which critical aspects of everyone's work is done simply enhances its total value and the meaningfulness of the experience to the child care workers.

As was indicated in chapter 2, the basic principles of child care work are the same either in the small setting or in the larger institution; the difference in the settings forces a difference in application. Child care theory as applied to the institutional care of children attempts to deal with some of those aspects of institutional living which differentiate it from day treatment and from treatment in the smaller residential center, and with those principles which have been developed as suitable guidelines for living and working in the larger setting. This discussion has introduced the child care worker to some of the administrative thinking which may underlie the working policies which are in effect. In understanding some of these background factors, the worker can more realistically and effectively perceive his own role and carry it out positively, so that he can best help achieve the goals of the institution and the therapeutic care of the children without sacrificing his own identity and convictions.

CHAPTER 11

The Individual Worker and the Staff

Communication

Chapter 3 describes the complicated process and meaning of the children's communication and the important role it plays in guiding the interaction between worker and child, as well as among the children themselves. The importance of intrastaff communication in the small treatment group in carrying out an effective treatment program for the children is underscored in chapter 6.

Clear and extensive communication takes on an even more basic importance when one considers the large number of people involved in maintaining the large institution and in executing different aspects of its program with the children. Cooperation and planning, coordination of approach, and integration of information all are required in handling treatment concerns of individual children and in developing the kind of program and milieu which will best promote the welfare of all the children. This cooperation is best achieved through comprehensive and effective methods of staff communication.

Two examples demonstrate the key role of communication in individual treatment and in total programming:

Jim, a ten-year-old boy, had been hospitalized for various kinds of acting-out behavior in the community and for the purpose of removing him from a chaotic and poorly supervised family situation. This boy was very cute in appearance and manner and had immediate appeal to everyone. The clinical staff knew that beyond his surface ability to charm was an inability to relate deeply to anyone. Rather, he was completely indiscriminate and would make the same friendly overtures to strangers that he would to those who were most closely involved in his care. These strangers among the other institutional personnel would often give him the material gratification that he usually requested—a coke, a candy bar, a nickel. However, a key part of his treatment program was to help him learn to develop relationships on a deeper basis and to find gratifications from contacts with people which did not always include giving him some material object or treat. Execution of this plan involved communicating to numerous persons the importance of not immediately succumbing to Jim's appealing manner by giving him a reward. It also included discussions with the supervisors of all the departments in the institution so that they could help their staffs with the difficult task of seeing that it was not really helping Jim for them to kid in front of him about how cute he was and to give him a nickel or a bar of candy.

The foregoing illustration shows the necessity of communication in the treatment of a single child. Communication is equally important in programming, an important vehicle for delivering treatment, the success of which depends on a smooth execution of the plans. An extensive network of communication is necessary so that all involved have been consulted about what is to take place and know what the program consists of; with whom, where, and when it will occur; and what the roles of each person involved are to be.

In one comprehensive institution serving a large number of children who had a variety of disabilities and were grouped by condition in large units in different buildings, it was felt that the unit team could best serve the needs of one of the boys on the unit by making an arrangement involving the children on another unit. A physically handicapped older boy who could read very well was to go to the unit of younger, withdrawn, emotionally disturbed boys to read to them. It was felt that this plan would benefit all involved. The boy, whose skill in reading was unusual in comparison to that of most of the other children and yet whose activities were limited because of his physical impairment, would have a chance to use his ability and thus increase his status and positive self-concept; the young boys would be provided with a new element of structure and stimulation in their daily program.

In order to implement this plan, the following communications were required: proposal of the program to the unit team of the younger boys' unit, arrangement with the education department to help select appropriate books for the reader's ability and the hearers' receptivity, arrangement with the transportation department to take the boy to and from the younger boys' unit, arrangement for an extra helper to accompany the boy since he was confined to a wheelchair, discussion with the supervisory nurse and the child care staff in each building to see that the boy would be ready to leave the one building and to be received in the other and to arrange for an appropriate area for the activity to take place, arrangement for specific staff to supervise the children while the activity was taking place, and finally informing the numerous people concerned what the specifics of the finalized plan were. Once the plan was worked out, it went smoothly, and the treatment goals around which it was developed were achieved, making, of course, everyone's efforts worthwhile.

Both of the above examples demonstrate how communication moves into the core of the treatment process in the large institution; coordinated communication is a must if the program is to run smoothly. Without communication people are confused and pass the confusion on to the children; programs are carried out haphazardly. Lack of communication and the resulting confusion are even more characteristic of institutions with the older type of staff organization. Under this system departments assign staff members to serve individual children living in various areas, and these staff members report on their work primarily to the sending department. Under that system the child's—and the staff's—experiences are often fragmented and confusing; departments often duplicate the efforts of others, omit some necessary services, and even unknowingly oppose one another. With the team approach, the staff members can have the kind of give-and-take which helps them to get to know one another and the ideas and approaches of the others, to understand one another's roles, and, most of all, to develop a feeling of working together to promote the children's optimal development in a situation in which the efforts of one team member complement and support those of the others.

For several reasons the development of a clear and comprehensive network of communication is one of the most complex tasks involved in running an institution. These reasons include the fact that it is usually impossible to get everybody who works with the children together at the same time. Since the children are in residence, somebody must always be responsible for providing direct supervision and thus cannot be present at a meeting. Also, since at least some of the children are present seven days a week, the child care staff assigned to any unit are not present every day since they have their days off. Furthermore, the shift system, which, of course, is necessary to provide round the clock care, means that the night shift is always off duty during the daytime hours when most of the clinical staff are on duty.

What procedures can and have been used to help all staff, particularly child care staff, give and receive the messages they need in order for the treatment program to progress smoothly?

The team meeting. One of the main vehicles for enhancing communication and the coordinated planning for the children's lives in the institution is the team approach. Originally employed to provide a treatment technique for smaller child-guidance centers and other agencies, this method is finding more and more application in the organization of larger institutions. The team approach involves the assigning of members of various disciplines to be responsible for planning and carrying out together the program and treatment for a specific group of children. Usually the children live in the same physical area of the institution, such as a cottage or wing of a building. Often a psychiatrist is the team leader, but sometimes it is a psychologist, social worker, professional child care worker, or nurse. Both through organized, planned, scheduled meetings and through more informal contacts as needed, the team members work together to achieve the overall goals for the children individually and as a group, each taking the role most appropriate for his training but tailoring his specific contribution to mesh with and enhance the work of the rest of the team.

The team meeting, which is a characteristic means of communication in institutions now employing the team approach, is often held once a week, with all those having contact with the particular group of children attending. At the meeting, programming, planning, and problems pertaining to both the individual children and the group as a whole are discussed.

The daily report. In some settings there are short daily meetings in which staff going on duty hear reports from staff going off about various occurrences and activities which have taken place. By understanding what has taken place since its last contact with the group, the new shift can better plan for and carry out the program. Thus carry-overs and continuations take place which would not have been possible otherwise. Such meetings are held at each change of shift.

Worker-organized meetings. Since time in the team meeting is limited and since the meeting must sometimes be focused on the management of individual children—on handling of acute behavior problems or on planning for the disposition of a child after he leaves the institution—the workers may feel that many matters which should be settled by the team are left undiscussed. In this case the workers can often arrange their own meetings, which can perhaps take place between shifts, with members of both shifts participating, and which can be used for planning group activities. The resulting plans can then be brought up briefly for approval at team meetings. Discussions can include such topics as trips and new ways of handling bedtime routines which are within the realm of the child care worker. This kind of initiative makes the worker very valuable to the institution and to the children, and supervisors may be pleased to allow time in the schedule for such meetings.

Daily notes. Since it is not possible for all messages to be conveyed verbally to everybody, the institution must make effective use of written communication, which can be made available to everybody. Child care workers are usually expected to write on some kind of behavior record form a summary of each child's behavior during their shift of duty. This is one area in which the child care worker can make a great contribution to everybody's knowledge and understanding of the child, and yet it is a task which it is tempting to pass off superficially at the end of an exhausting day with the children. Instead of trying to recapitulate the highlights of each child's behavior for the day, the worker may fall back on such blanket phrases as "good day," "poor day," "hyper," "quiet," "usual self." A cycle is set up in which nobody reads the notes because there is nothing in them and nobody writes extensive notes because nobody reads them. Perceptive, thoughtful daily notations on each individual child will prove to be of real use to all who deal with the children. To draw attention of other staff to his notes, a worker might say at a meeting, for example, "I have put some other examples of this kind of behavior from Johnny in my ward notes." Summaries of daily notes and reports of work with the child by other disciplines and agencies are placed in the child's permanent file, which is usually kept in a central area of the institution.

The communication book.   Aside from individual clinical records on the children, there are other modes of written communication which are or perhaps should be employed in the large institution, since they are potentially effective ways of enhancing program coordination and smooth functioning of the living unit. One of the most useful of these is a notebook called a "communication book," which is kept in a central spot, such as the nursing station, readily accessible to anyone coming onto the unit. In it messages are recorded by anyone having something relevant to communicate. A typical day's entries might include, for example, the details of plans for an outing, the time and date of the next staff meeting, the fact that a certain child is upset because of a piece of bad news from home, a note that the drinking fountain is now repaired, a reminder that Johnny must be taken for an eye exam at 2:30, and what the new policy is about children's keeping food in their rooms. This type of message must be relayed to all, and the communication book is an effective way of doing it.

The policy book.   Some institutions have policy books which are available to all the staff and describe the unit's basic procedures for handling the various aspects of the program and the routines of daily living. These can be most helpful, if they are kept up-to-date, particularly to new and relief staff. With such a book to orient them to the way things are done on the unit, staff members are not left in a quandary when children tell them, "Oh, the regular workers let us go to bed at ten o'clock," "We don't have to wear sweaters outside unless we want to," etc. The knowledge of unit policy gained from the book gives the worker firm ground upon which to stand.

The bulletin board. Bulletin boards for posting the daily schedule of each child have been instituted in some settings. Clever workers can devise ways of indicating each department's activity and the time of the activity, as well as ways of readily making changes in the master schedule as the child's program changes. Tape, thumbtacks, different colors of construction paper, etc., can be used by the workers to devise an effective daily schedule board. It is helpful if this board is kept in a location where both staff and children can use it. Access to such a schedule helps the children to develop a conception of the structure and passage of time and to feel a sense of order and predictability in their lives.

Staff Relationships

As has been pointed out in previous sections of this book, it is realized nowadays that the quality of intrastaff relationships is a key factor in determining the overall quality of the child's treatment program. In the institution, where the work may at times be stressful and frustrating and where there are many people with individual orientations and personalities, staff disagreements can crop up. Yet in the institution it is important that every possible positive resource be brought to bear to contribute to the children's treatment program, and thus it is crucial that staff relationships be smooth and comfortable so far as possible. This section discusses some specific aspects of the relationships of the child care worker to the rest of the institutional personnel, describes some of the typical problems that can occur, and suggests what in some instances can contribute toward their resolution.

Supervisors. The relationship between the child care workers and their immediate supervisor is among the most important. In the large institution, as in most child care settings of any size, the workers are under the supervision of a senior staff member, whose training may be in any one of a number of disciplines such as nursing, professional child care, social work, education, and psychology. The type of discipline represented by the supervisor depends on the availability of staff and on the overall administrative conception and philosophy of the institution. For example, in the children's treatment unit of a large hospital, the basic structure is probably a medical one and the immediate supervisor is a nurse. Some residential "schools" carry over their teaching orientation into the twenty-four-hour-a-day living situation; thus supervisors are sometimes teachers. Professional child care workers with graduate study in child care are not yet numerous, but when there is one available, he or she is likely to be a supervisor of child care workers.

Individual supervisors have different styles, different ways of fulfilling this overall function. Sometimes the supervisor may establish a climate in which the children are encouraged to develop their deepest, their "prime" relationships with the child care workers. He performs many background administrative duties which provide the workers with the opportunity to give to the children both emotionally and materially, and he may even do some of the unit chores now and then so that more of the workers' time is freed for them to be right with the children. The supervisor tries to stay out of the way and to leave both the authority and the relationship with the children to the workers. He supports the workers, to help them do what they collectively think is best for the children. Another, less usual style of supervision is that in which the supervisor establishes close, therapeutic relationships with every child and encourages the children to work their problems out with him. The child care workers are encouraged to develop wholesome, but not intensive, relationships with the children within a framework of programming and physical care. In some settings there is a combination of these approaches, with the supervisor developing close relationships with some of the children and yet also spending part of his time and effort in developing the unit climate so that the workers may relate to others, according to the inclination of the children to gravitate toward one adult or another.

Especially when a supervisor uses the first style, the workers may sometimes realize that they are "better with the children" than the supervisor is. This is natural enough. Now that there are some training courses in child care and the institutions are recognizing their value, some of the unit workers may have had intensive training; other workers may have high aptitude and/or long experience. The unit supervisor may have had very little specific training in child care but may be trained in a related field. When a supervisor deliberately keeps himself in the background so that the children may relate to the workers, the children naturally feel closer to the workers, just as schoolchildren feel closer to their teachers than they do to the principal. The children may even select the supervisor as the person on whom to take out their anger for what they dislike about the institution. The worker should not fall into the trap of supporting this attitude, however, but should let the children know that the supervisor is responsible for helping them have good times as well as for initiating and backing up the rules which they may not like so much, but which are instituted for their own growth and safety.

The support of the supervisor is necessary if the worker is to do a good job. The worker should learn to use his part of the supervisory relationship in such a way as to enhance his own work. The supervisor has overall responsibility for the unit. He can mobilize and coordinate the resources of the institution in such a way as to help make the worker's efforts fruitful.

Fellow workers. Among child care workers themselves, the major sources of disagreement aside from various day-to-day stresses are variations in individual attitudes and practices toward discipline, housekeeping, etc. This discord often occurs between shifts. Workers who have been together for a while often develop a cohesiveness among themselves. They have worked out a comfortable division of labor, and the exigencies of the work, with the occasional crises, have served to draw them together. Thus whatever they feel is wrong within the area of child care responsibilities they are tempted to see as the fault of another shift. If a supervisor criticizes the housekeeping on the unit, the evening shift may say, "Well, the 7:00 to 3:00 shift never cleans up after the children have been playing"; or if the teachers say the children are coming to school tired, the 7:00 to 3:00 shift may say, "Oh, the 3:00 to 11:00 shift just lets them watch television for half the night."

A supervisor was confronted by a situation of this kind in which at the time of the shift change a child coming in from school asked for paper to start his homework. The evening worker said, "It's not 3:30 [his time to come on formal duty] yet, so the day shift should set it out for you." The day workers were finishing up their reports in the office and did not want to take care of the child's request either, since they thought they were through for the day. The supervisor helped the child, then spoke with both shifts about the key issue, which was attending to the child's needs rather than making it a petty shift contention, which undermined the child's confidence in *all* the workers, since he had to stand around listening while they argued about who was going to take care of him.

Other disciplines. A similar type of difficulty sometimes develops between child care workers and members of other disciplines when they are working with a group of children simultaneously. Each set of workers feels that there are some things which it should not do because they are "OT's job," "the child care workers' job," "the recreation workers' job," etc. Thus activity workers may feel that they should not change a child's diaper while they are working with him; the child care worker may feel that he does not need to plan any activities for the children because that is the activity worker's job.

Another type of problem in relationships between child care workers and other departments is centered in the general area of discipline. Child care staffs often feel angry at other staffs who allow the children freedoms which they are not able to permit, especially if the workers have to clean up or deal with the results of the incident, such as having to take away from a child a cigarette given him by another staff member. Child care workers often feel that they have the most difficult job with the children and yet have the fewest tools available to help them control the children. Thus they sometimes want to be able to deny the child an activity offered by another department as a consequence of the child's misbehaving while in the care of the worker. If the worker keeps the child back from the activity, the offering department often resents this action.

In one institution a method of handling this situation which was agreeable to all was devised. If the child care worker felt that a child's behavior necessitated his being kept back from an activity, he would discuss his feelings with the supervisor, without saying anything to the child. Usually the supervisor could see that the worker's feelings were justified; if he did not, he would explain his reasons in terms of the child's overall treatment plan. The supervisor would then contact the other department to discuss the matter and devise a mutually acceptable plan. The child care worker could then tell the child what the plans would be for him regarding his attendance at the next activity, thus upholding his own authority with the child and yet avoiding conflict with the other department.

Therapists. In settings where the children are receiving individual therapy, the relationship between the child care worker and the individual therapist is another one to consider. The therapist, realizing the importance of the worker's daily close contacts with the children, generally asks him about what has been going on in the child's life. This knowledge provides the therapist with significant information which he needs to carry out the most effective treatment with the child. Conversely, many therapists share the important occurrences in the child's sessions with the workers. If this is done, it contributes to an effective give-and-take between the individuals involved. On the other hand, some therapists feel that their exchanges with the children should be confidential, or they feel certain cases should be. There are some children who must have assurance that nobody else will know what goes on in their sessions if they are to participate fully and get the benefit that is intended from them. In this case the worker may feel that his brains are constantly being picked and that he gets no feedback. But this lack of communication may be necessary at times and in no way detracts from the value of what the worker does.

The contact between worker and therapist involves not just the exchange of information but the possibility of a deeper assessment of the child's development and needs. The therapist can be of assistance to the worker in helping to explain the underlying reasons for some of the child's behavior and in helping the worker to feel more secure in what he is doing in the face of what often is incomprehensible behavior. The therapist may not always be able to tell the worker how to respond to a given kind of behavior, but he can often enlighten the worker as to its meaning and help him explore ways of managing it. Sometimes therapists do offer suggestions for management and handling of the child in the daily living situation which they feel will help support the goals that are being worked on in therapy. Usually it is in the child's best interest for the workers to make an effort to carry them out, because the therapist is often able to point out needs of which other staff are unaware. Occasionally, however, the measures which the therapist requests are not compatible with some of the principles of the unit program. In such a case, if the worker can explain the problem, the therapist may be able to modify his suggestions so that everyone is satisfied. In case of a strong difference of opinion, the unit supervisor may be able to work out a compromise.

The child care worker may notice that the type of relationship that he observes between a therapist and the child is different from the one that he has. Sometimes the child may seem to be on his worst behavior in the therapist's presence. This is often due to the fact that at certain points in therapy problem areas are deliberately opened up so that they can be worked on. Thus the worker may observe more symptomatic behavior in the child before and/or after a therapy session. At other times the child may seem extremely fond of and dependent on the therapist. He may say to the worker, "I'll only tell my therapist about that." The worker may feel resentful at this attachment. However, it may be very important that the child have this relationship in order to get better. The worker should also understand that the child cannot get better without the different but crucial support and understanding of the worker.

Administration. Although in some large settings workers do not have frequent contact with the unit director and head administrator—usually a medically trained person, a psychiatrist or pediatrician—this trend is changing now that the importance of the child care function is increasingly recognized. More and more, the worker will find himself being asked about the behavior of specific children on the unit and also being asked to contribute his suggestions and opinions regarding changes and innovations in the program and in the living units. When the workers' contribution to the treatment of the children is given this positive regard, the workers themselves are better motivated to do a good job and to tolerate the inevitable frustrations of their duties, realizing that without their best service the children's lives would be much less rich. When the workers can identify with the administrator of the unit, they avoid the development of the resentful attitude, "If they spent as much time with the youngsters as we do, things might be done differently around here."

Handling relationships. No matter how benign and sympathetic the administrators and supervisors of an institution are, no matter how effective the communications system is, and no matter how much importance is attached to the role of the child care worker, inevitably there will be times when the individual worker finds himself angry at another person. Because so many people of varying orientation and personality are involved with the children and because of the nature of the work, it is impossible for all stresses among the staff to be prevented. Thus the child care worker will encounter situations which make him sufficiently annoyed that he will feel like taking action. Chapter 6 discusses the handling of one's feelings in the smaller setting; the feelings of the worker in the institution are not different, but his situation is more complicated.

First of all, it is important to underscore again the reasons for the workers' attempts to manage their feelings in an adult fashion.

Studies have shown that staff dissension in treatment settings for mental illness is almost directly reflected in the behavior of the patients. Thus the children inevitably tune into staff squabbles and behave in ways which are more difficult for everyone to handle, and this situation, of course, detracts from the success of the treatment.

In a new unit in an institution, two supervisors of different backgrounds but with joint responsibility for the supervision of child care workers on this unit did not agree on the type of duties which the workers should emphasize. On some days one supervisor would come on duty earlier than the other. When the other supervisor would arrive, he would notice a negative and almost hostile attitude on the part of the children which was not observable on other days when the first supervisor was off duty or had not yet come on. The conflicting emphases of the two senior staff members were confusing to the child care workers, who, having been guided earlier in the day by one supervisor, then felt resentful when the other one came on. The children had no trouble perceiving this confusion and readily showed it in their behavior.

The worker may remember from his own family experience or that of his friends how children feel when they are present at parental quarrels or are made aware of more than routine disagreements. Children in institutions have similar feelings when they see those in charge not getting along.

Not all conflicts of opinions can be worked out; nor is it necessary that they should be. It is necessary only that both points of view be recognized and that a plan of action somehow be worked out. The team meeting is one place in which the worker can express his concerns. Sincere differences of opinion expressed without animosity about the overall program or about an individual child are suitable to bring up for staff consideration at a team meeting, and often the other staff can offer alternative plans, suggestions, and support. However, person-to-person gripes are not always most appropriately worked out in a group meeting—it depends upon the nature of the meeting. In some institutions meetings for just this purpose are set up under the leadership of someone trained in group dynamics. Otherwise it may be better for the two parties who disagree to meet together with the unit supervisor.

Similar policy should be the guideline for use of the communication book. Notes specifically aimed at criticizing another person serve only to generate and snowball angry feelings rather than to solve the problems causing the worker to feel upset.

The worker can learn to express himself tactfully, in a way that can convey his concern without reflecting publicly upon somebody else. If he is annoyed because one child care worker, Mike, has been leaving doors unlocked, he can say, "I wonder if we should all go over the policy for locking doors," rather than "Mike is always leaving doors unlocked, and I'm the one who has to go after the children when they discover this." Or if another worker, Jane, has been giving the children money when this is not permitted, another worker might say, "Can we talk about the effect on a child when he gets money from just one or two of us?" The offending worker usually understands the implications from what is said, but this presentation of the issue prevents real hostility from developing.

Another resource for the worker to employ in dealing with such concerns is the unit supervisor. Some supervisors are able to and are in a position to correct disturbing situations in such a way that sensitive feelings are spared. And of course, he has the authority to make changes that the worker may not have. Most supervisors want to know what is bothering the workers and often indicate that their doors are open for private discussions with the workers concerning problems on the unit. This availability is important, for many times just being able to talk out a problem helps the worker restore his equilibrium. The supervisor can sometimes take steps to smooth over a difficult situation between staff members which please both and also do not sacrifice the children's care.

In a unit housing a large number of hyperactive children, one child who was very attractive was also a problem for the workers to manage, showing much self-destructive behavior. One day activity workers assigned to the unit came to the supervisor in anger, saying that the unit child care workers were cruel because they had asked the nurse to put the child in isolation for a while. The supervisor found out upon investigation that the child was especially hard to manage that day and also that one regular worker was away. He also discovered that the activity workers' real concern was that the child would become even more self-destructive since he would have nothing to do in isolation. The supervisor was able to work out a compromise which respected both positions. He could understand the need of the child care workers to be relieved temporarily of the supervision of the child, and he could also agree with the feelings of the activity workers that the child needed occupation to prevent his behavior from becoming worse. He thus worked out an arrangement for the child to remain in isolation but to be provided with a comfortable chair and some safe activities, with the activity workers spending some time with him to help him with the activities and provide human contact.

Probably one of the best philosophical guidelines to be offered to the worker in handling his feelings is that of a wise psychiatrist who served in promoting the creation of a positive climate in an institution. She recommended that in any instance of dissension, the focus should be on the welfare of *the child,* rather than on the faults, omissions, or personalities of the staff. When staff members consider their gripes from this point of view, they soon find themselves seeking together positive solutions for the problems of the children, rather than becoming divided by their individual contrary feelings.

In the period before a team meeting in a large institution, feelings were at a high pitch between some of the workers. One group thought that Jimmy was being allowed too much freedom by the others and should be isolated more frequently. The other group felt that it was important for Jimmy to have the kind of freedom that they were permitting him. As soon as the meeting began, workers from both factions began talking loudly about their concerns. Rather than taking a stand as to who was right and who was wrong, the doctor went over Jimmy's history before entering the institution. This review enabled both sides to see their behavior in a different perspective, without being put on the spot, and soon an approach was developed which was best for Jimmy and which made sense to all.

Conclusions

The various chapters of Part III have enumerated and examined some of the aspects of the challenging and fascinating job of institutional child care. It has been pointed out in honesty that there are some difficulties indigenous to work in such a setting, so that the worker going into the institution may not be unduly shaken by what he encounters and so that he may have the background and understanding to function most effectively. This part has also pointed out what the advantages of the institution are in providing good care and treatment for the child and, most specifically, what the many opportunities are for the child care worker to make a real contribution toward developing a therapeutic and growth-producing environment for the children.

The child care worker is an important element in the new orientation in institutional settings toward giving treatment and not just custodial care. Concomitant with the gradual elevation of the role and status of child care and its practitioners, there have been changes in ideas about what might constitute effective treatment for disturbed children. Some of these more recent ideas demand exactly those unique competencies which the trained child care worker possesses.

Formerly it was felt that the primary treatment of children occurred only in individual therapy sessions and that the institution and workers existed to house the children and to provide physical care and protection while they waited for their treatment hour to roll around. Nowadays it is realized by almost everyone that while individual therapy is certainly important and in some cases really necessary for the children's improvement, the remainder of the time, when the child care workers are in charge, is also crucially important in determining the course of the children's progress.

It was once felt that in order for a disturbed child to recover, it was necessary for his earliest stages of development to be relived and retraced through intensive therapy. Again this idea is unfeasible in terms not only of time and expense but of its unsuitability for many children. Fortunately, the great value of a somewhat different approach has been recognized recently; it is one which is readily applicable to the setting of a large institution. This is a child-development philosophy, an environmental style of treatment which attempts to discover where the child is on a continuum of growth and development and consequently to tailor that environment in an increasingly challenging fashion to the child's force for growth. He is provided with the kind of program that builds upon his strengths and makes restitution in areas where his development is lacking. The components of such an environment include a rich diet of educational and recreational activities, a wholesome pattern of daily living, the opportunity to develop gratifying relationships with other children and adults, and the understanding of each child's individual needs. The child care worker in the large institution can play a key role in providing these ingredients for positive development.

PART IV

Activity Programming

by Karen Dahlberg VanderVen

Developmental Programming
for the Worker

Elements of Activity Programming

Many talented and sensitive workers show an understanding of the dynamics of children's behavior and of the various ways in which the children in their care communicate. These workers are able to respond appropriately to many of the children's emotional needs, to resolve "crisis" situations, to develop close and meaningful relationships with the children. All of these things are, of course, essential in providing fine clinical child care.

So that these interpersonal skills may be most effectively brought to bear in the task of providing therapeutic care, another tool in the child care worker's bag of tricks is also essential: knowledge of activity programming. In essence, this is practical know-how on "what to do" with children and what to have them do during the many hours when the worker is responsible for them, hours in which they are not occupied by another specific routine of daily living or by school or therapy sessions. It allows the worker to set the stage and supply the props for the important work he does in helping the children deal with their feelings and relationships. A worker cannot discuss the children's anger if they are running helter-skelter; he cannot even get them together. Children's expression of feelings of boredom can be sympathetically acknowledged and accepted, but if there is a real basis to them, the children will not get better just by having their feelings accepted. The withdrawn children cannot be helped to relate to one another just through talking, at least at first; they need to be doing something together.

These are just a few of the kinds of situations that the child care worker will encounter frequently—situations in which he must both manage the children and promote the kind of therapeutic climate which helps them develop. To deal with these situations, the worker needs two things: his theoretical or intuitive understanding of the dynamics and feelings of the children and also, on the practical level, skills in activity programming. With this knowledge the worker has some means for drawing an active group together. With it he can prevent the children from becoming bored much of the time. He can involve the withdrawn children in an interesting activity that will help them notice one another.

This chapter deals with activity programming for the child care worker, its special function in the worker's repertoire of skills and in the children's treatment, and ways in which the worker can most effectively select and conduct activities to meet the children's needs. Specific activities will not be described extensively. It is assumed that the worker will be familiar from his own childhood and life experiences with the content or techniques involved in conducting the activity, or that they can easily be learned from books or discussions with other workers. This chapter focuses on a more difficult task for the worker—understanding the importance of activities and knowing how to plan and conduct them to meet the overall treatment goals of individuals and groups.

Programming is part of the responsibility of the child care worker in a setting of any size although its function in the treatment of the children, the pattern of its execution, and the part of the child care worker in carrying it out vary from setting to setting. Before examining in detail the many aspects of effective program planning, it will be helpful to spell out some ways in which the worker might be involved in it.

As was pointed out in chapter 7, in a large setting, such as a state institution, many activities might be provided by separate departments or disciplines on a somewhat formal, scheduled basis.

In this arrangement children are taken to another area of the institution for program. In some instances the practice has been for the child care workers not to participate, either staying on their units to do housekeeping chores or possibly sitting on the sideline of the acitvity until the children are through. (As we shall see, it is far more beneficial for the workers to join in the activity rather than to watch or otherwise be involved.) Even if this is the predominant programming model in a setting, however, the workers have many hours when the children *are* on the unit "unprogrammed" by other departments, for which they must take the initiative with such activities as they can plan. So that these times can be pleasant and productive, it is important that the workers take this initiative. Many feel that this general type of programming for children is not the most effective: it fragments staff efforts. Communication is difficult, so that workers in one area may lack important information from another which would help them in planning a coordinated program meaningful to the children in its totality. Goals and purposes may be misconstrued, so that staff friction is more likely to develop. Finally, to the children the view of staff is a fragmented one too; they see people and activities as belonging to separate areas, rather than working together. Some institutions get around some of the difficulties inherent in this plan by using "activity coordinators" to help the various departments coordinate and relate their efforts, but even with this help close planning and communication may be difficult.

In other settings, usually those in which a team approach is employed, the child care workers may have a broader job in activity programming. They participate in the overall planning of activities and accompany the children on their off-unit activities. After the initial discussion, the final plan and the materials may be supplied by the activity department, with the workers helping the departmental staff to carry out the activities directly with the children. This type of structure is the most effective if used carefully. The workers' special knowledge of the children's individual ways of responding, their commitment (hopefully!) to the value of the activity for the children, and their "helping hands" aid each child to participate as fully as possible. Also, the children have an opportunity to relate to the staff in a different way from the way they relate on the living unit. And, of course, communication is enhanced among the staff; each department understands better what the other is doing and each learns from the other. Even when child care workers do join other departments in activities, however, there are again times when the workers must provide constructive program on the unit without the direction of another discipline. Usually, their experience with jointly programmed activities gives them further resources and enthusiasm for their own on-unit activities; highly motivated workers may even request that other departments give them suggestions and directions for appropriate activities.

In some very small settings, finally, the child care worker might be responsible for the program content of the child's entire day, even, in some agencies, for his educational programming. Here the worker must not only carry out each activity but select activities for various times during the day which can serve a variety of goals and which provide a balance in the child's life. For example, one activity may be primarily educational in the academic sense and another more recreational—although in the treatment of disturbed children there is a special educational component in any carefully planned activity. In this arrangement, of course, communication and coordination problems are minimized; the possible drawback is that enrichment and variety may be lost unless workers make a concerted and energetic effort in program-planning.

The child care worker's awareness of the crucial function of program in the broad area of therapeutic developmental care and his knowledge and skills in programming will, in any situation, play a key part in determining whether his and even others' time with the children—no matter how long and with how many—will be fraught with boredom, purposelessness, and exaggeratedly symptomatic behavior or whether his sojourn will be productive, if not always tranquil. No matter who is directly responsible for doing it, activity programming is not a simple matter of laying out a few materials and letting the children loose. It involves considerable effort on the part of the worker. Execution of a programmed activity involves the following elements:

1. Choosing the type of activity that will be appropriate for a specific period of time, given the particular individual and group needs at the time
2. Determining what materials and equipment will be needed
3. Selecting an appropriate physical setting in which to carry out the activity
4. Anticipating possible behavioral reactions to the activity and ways in which they might be handled
5. Determining what the type of involvement in the activity will be for both children and adults.

For example, we may come onto a unit of disturbed children and note that they seem to be casually painting. When we look beneath the surface, however, there has been much more taking place, as we can see when we consider the activity in terms of the four elements just cited: first of all, the workers selected painting for the children because they had just returned from an active ball game with recreational workers and a quiet activity seemed indicated. Having decided on painting, the workers then needed to ascertain where the best place on the unit would be to conduct the activity. Since this unit had a room for "messy" activities, this was easily picked as the appropriate area. Their job was not done, however, for they still needed to present the art materials in such a way that, for example, each child had enough paint so that there would not have to be too much sharing in a group that was not yet able to do this. Individual reactions were also considered: what would the workers do if Johnny characteristically refused to participate or if Jimmy spilled the paint? Workers also were concerned with what the cues would be for stopping the activity before the children, having tired of it, began to splash over their paintings. Finally the workers thought about who should stand by Johnny to to give him the special guidance he would need to participate in this kind of activity, who would be in charge of making sure that each person had enough materials, who would be involved in cleaning up. Hardly a simple situation after all, but it is one in which, as a result of special efforts made to conduct it effectively, growth will take place.

How Programming Helps the Children

Now that some of the elements involved in programming have been outlined, we can look at some of the reasons for making the concerted effort required for effective programming. What indeed are the specific therapeutic benefits for the children? And how does programming help busy staff achieve their challenging task of promoting the children's overall welfare and development while it helps them to "manage" their charges as well?

Developmental Aspects of Programming

The major function of programming is to enhance the children's development. Simply stated, this means that the children's activity program, when it is carefully designed and carried out as an integral part of their daily lives, plays an essential role in providing the kinds of experiences which promote their overall development. Among the more specific areas of development supported by good activity program are education, self-expression, self-esteem, and socialization.

Educational function. Experts in the treatment of disturbed children are becoming increasingly aware of the importance of programming in achieving treatment goals. Not only do disturbed children need, so far as possible, to pick up previously missed stages of development but as part of this process they also need reeducation and exposure to those types of learning experiences which normal children have. In other words, they need to learn about the "reality" of the world and how to deal with and react to it as other people do. The direction, the content, and the patterned stimulation provided through activity programming help serve this essential function of helping the children to learn to understand and deal with aspects of the real world. The psychological characteristics necessary for this understanding to take place are called ego-functions. Disturbed children, as has already been said, are deficient in the development of many ego-functions which normal children gradually acquire in the course of their growth. Many ego-functions have been studied by psychologists;

most of them can be stimulated toward development and expression through activity programming. Although it is not within the scope of this chapter to relate the various ego-functions to specific activities, we can examine a few of them, such as awareness of the capacities of one's body (body image), perceptual ability, capacity to experience pleasure, and ability to tolerate frustration.

Most disturbed children are not aware of their basic physical abilities or else hold a distorted view of their bodies in relationship to their environment. Their sense of themselves is inadequate. Activity program supports in many ways the development of an increased awareness in the children of what they can do with their bodies. When they learn, through the initiative and guidance of their child care workers, to throw a ball, to control a paintbrush, or to push a saw back and forth, they are increasing their ability to use their bodies effectively toward the accomplishment of a realistic task and thus increasing also their own self-awareness.

A major deficit in many disturbed children is in the ability to organize the input of stimulation received from the environment. They cannot use their sensory apparatus to give them a realistic view of what is going on around them. Through activities which require that children use their eyes and ears, even their noses and mouths—in coordination with other parts of their bodies—for a specific purpose, they are helped to develop this essential ability to integrate the stimulation they receive from their surroundings. Activities indeed offer organized sensory stimulation and provide situations in which children can begin to feel comfortable in allowing new perceptions into their experience.

Normal adults who are accustomed to enjoying many pleasures in life and recall similarly happy experiences from their own childhood are amazed when they see disturbed children who in general seem to take little if any pleasure in the kinds of experience which normal children find delightful. For example, a disturbed child may be apathetic at his own birthday party and give his special present only a passing glance and touch. Through constant and consistent exposure to carefully planned activities, children gradually acquire the ego-function of the capacity to experience pleasure.

As a final example we can consider the ability to tolerate frustration. This, of course, is a major deficit in the behavioral repertoire of disturbed children. Workers see some children react intensely to the slightest annoyance; they may abandon an effort at the first snag. Activity programming helps them gradually to increase their controls—for example, the model plane that the worker helps a boy to build engages the child's interest so much that he does not throw on the floor the freshly glued piece which slips out of place but rather replaces it.

These four ego-functions have been cited as illustrations to indicate to the worker how his efforts to expose his charges to activities in doses which they can handle can contribute toward essential areas in their overall development. As they are helped, through activities, to develop basic ego-functions, they then become accessible to further educational experiences.

Expressive function.   In addition to their inability to interpret reality, disturbed children also have problems, as was pointed out in chapter 3, in expressing their feelings, some even in knowing *what* they are feeling. It is a prime function of the child care worker (along with the rest of the treatment team) to help each child come to understand his feelings better and to be able to express them more appropriately. If, for example, a child has come to realize that he feels anger, he must gradually learn that when he is angry, the acceptable way to handle this feeling is to talk about it and not to hurl the nearest object at the closest person.

Activities can help a child achieve this most important task of mastering his feelings. To learn how he feels, he must be exposed to situations which elicit reactions from him. Activities can provide many of these situations; here a worker can, through talking and working with the child, help him to see what feelings are involved.

A worker was having a biweekly activity session with a very withdrawn seven-year-old boy. The goal of the sessions was to help him, through the activities selected, to develop more awareness of his body and, most particularly, to encourage him to use his strength, which he seemed reluctant to use. If he had a ball, he would aimlessly drop it rather than throw it. If swimming, he would let his legs dangle, rather than kick. For a while, in his activity sessions he would hold a saw inserted in a piece of wood but would not push it. The worker gradually but persistently encouraged him to use his full arm strength to push the saw back and forth. This made the boy angry, and at first he would only push the saw appropriately when he was feeling angry. This situation helped to bring out both this child's reluctance to use his strength and his feelings of anger, so they could be dealt with by both child and worker. Without the activity medium of saw and wood, which comprised an area for working through these particular feelings, this important learning could not have taken place.

As the child learns to recognize his feelings, he also needs appropriate means through which to express them. As activities can help a child learn about his feelings through eliciting his reactions around certain situations, so they can provide him with a suitable channel through which to express them. With normal children observers have noted some of the relationships between feelings about various developmental tasks and the opportunity to master these feelings through play with certain kinds of materials. For example, children with concern about toileting often find comfort—and mastery of feelings—through play with clay and water. Through various activities disturbed children can do the same thing. Feelings of anger can be drained off through active games and through crafts involving hammering and pounding. Fears can be expressed through symbolic play with dolls, models, and other materials which allow for dramatic play. And, as one authority has summed it up, to overcome a fear of, say, playing ball, a child must do more than simply talk about the fear in therapy. He must have the chance to play ball to master his fear. It is this ball game which the child care worker can provide.

Self-esteem and positive self-concept.   If one could summarize in one concept the main problems of disturbed children, he would not be far off in saying that it would center around the lack of positive self-concept—of awareness of oneself as a person of value, even in some cases of who one is and where he stands in relationship to others and the world at large. Through previous lack of stimulation, through upbringing—in some cases within a distorted family structure—or through inability for reasons we do not understand to capitalize on the experiences which help normal children progress in their development, disturbed children often lack in one way or another the crucial sense of who they are; or if they have a self-concept, it often seems negative, for example, they feel, "I'm a bad boy." It is difficult for workers to develop a feeling for such highly disturbed children as people.

Through activity programming many of the deficits which contribute to the child's lack of positive self-concept can be restored; also as the workers observe the children beginning to respond, they become better able to regard the children positively. How both of these outcomes are achieved can perhaps be best shown through examples:

After eight-year-old Artie, a severely disturbed nonverbal boy, had been exposed to music through song time on his treatment unit, he learned to sing "Row, Row, Row Your Boat." Since he had never responded to anything so positively, this achievement gave the workers great pleasure and they often asked him to sing it. Realizing the warm response he could evoke, he would sing with obvious pleasure, and as time went on this one new ability spearheaded development of others. As a result, he began to look upon himself more positively, and much of the self-punitive behavior he had shown before his first achievement was made decreased.

Another severely disturbed boy, Jack, spent much spare time compulsively manipulating small objects he picked up around the unit. Workers began asking him to help them with legitimate "picking up" tasks which, because of his original propensities, he was able to perform well. His achievement gave him a brand new image in the eyes of the workers, who then saw him as a real helper, rather than as a child who only indulged in meaningless activity, and the relationships between the child and the workers became more positive.

It should be pointed out, of course, that activities are not a cure-all in and of themselves; nor are they the only way in which disturbed children develop self-esteem. Within the context of a therapeutic environment, however, activity programming does make a significant contribution in helping children feel better about themselves.

Socialization. Doing things according to plans, or in ways encouraged by other people, or with other people, as is the case with activities, offers an ideal means for developing socialized behavior. With highly withdrawn children it is difficult for workers to know how to establish contact in order to begin to develop a relationship. How do you approach a child who wants to spin a wheel in his fingers for hours uninterrupted by anyone? What do you say to a child who tells you to "get out of here, you—" when you approach him? The framework for interaction provided by activities helps workers to handle these situations constructively. If a worker can say to either child, "We're going to play some records now," he has some means around which to structure interaction between himself and the child. Even if the children resist or act negatively, they and the worker have something to talk about. The withdrawn child may continue to spin, and the acting-out one may say, "I don't want to play no records," but still the worker's comment is facilitating interaction. In other words, an important way to gain an entry into social interaction with a disturbed child is to approach him about participation in an activity.

The activities help staff and children to share reality, and this association, through the staff's own understanding of the elements involved, can help the children focus their feelings about the experience they are having. Look at the negative social behavior and feelings among children and staff in one instance when there was no unifying activity taking place:

Two workers sat at a table in the middle of the room, smoking and chatting. In one corner a verbal child was subtly provoking a more withdrawn one, poking him in the hope that his symptomatic behavior, biting his wrist, would then emerge so he could make fun of him. One more withdrawn child was sitting in another corner, rocking back and forth on his haunches. Another child, an anxious although verbal one, would occasionally try to dart out of the room. When a worker became aware of what was taking place behind his back, he would shout, "Get back in here!"

It is obvious that this situation was hardly a healthy one for anybody involved; neither children nor workers were learning to live with one another or understand one another better. This is not to say, of course, that there must be a constant beehive of activity; planned hiatuses can be most fruitful. Rather, it is to point out that an activity can provide the means to encourage socialized behavior among children who otherwise would be hard to reach. We can contrast the anecdote above with the following incident:

Two workers and five severely disturbed children were sitting around a table making decorations for a forthcoming open house. Larry, who usually did not do much, nonetheless had just followed the worker's instructions to drop glitter in a glued area. One of the workers said to the other with obvious pleasure, "Hey, look what Larry just did!" Two verbal children at one end of the table who had never had much to do with each other and had not had much positive experience in sharing had to share the glue. The basic pleasure experienced in this situation where workers and children were having a positive association "caught" these children and soon they were very politely asking each other, "Can I use the glue now, Bob?" and, "Sure, I'm done now, Tom." Later, when the activity was taping the decorations on the wall, Bob and Tom, having helped each other by holding a picture while the other taped, then spontaneously began helping the younger withdrawn children. All the children seemed to respond positively to the new kinds of interaction stimulated through their joint participation in this activity.

Another crucial way in which activity programming can contribute to the socialization of disturbed children is to provide them with typical childhood experiences which normal children in the community automatically receive in the process of growing up. For children who are unable to live in the community or do not have the individual capacity to initiate typical games and activities with other children, an important part of development can be missed. Restitution to the children of these missed experiences can be an important contribution of the child care worker. If one looks back to his own childhood—as one inevitably does in the course of working with children—he can remember the many hours spent playing games with one's peers—cards, board games, games of skill such as jacks, and active games such as Hide-and-Seek. One can remember making lanyards, plaster of Paris statues, and other craft projects. The significance of these memories is obvious. They show the universality among children of certain kinds of activities which have been shared and passed along to one another for years. Workers from different localities and even of different age groups on exchanging notes will find that they have participated in many of the same kinds of activities. Writers on child development call this shared tradition of play among children "the culture of middle years." Its relevance to our discussion here is again to underscore the importance of stimulating this kind of experience for disturbed children who are out of the mainstream of this culture. The worker must serve as a surrogate of children's culture, bringing these experiences directly to those in his care and presenting them in such a way that the children can make them part of their understanding of the world.

Thus the worker can see how his initiative in planning and stimulating activity can serve numerous important treatment goals for the child, as well as develop a climate of vitality and involvement which makes life together more enjoyable and interesting for all concerned. This is especially important in large institutions where, as was pointed out in chapter 7, the workers' efforts around providing program comprise a significant component of the entire treatment plan.

Observation and Diagnosis

Previous chapters have cited the importance of the child care worker as an observer of significant aspects of a child's behavior which others who do not spend as much time with him may never have the opportunity to see. When the children are essentially unoccupied, workers, indeed, get a chance to see what the children do under such circumstances. But when the children are involved in programmed activities, workers are given specialized situations in which to observe their reactions.

For example, some activities inevitably contain the option for success or failure: you catch or drop the ball, saw on a straight or a crooked line, put the right amount of milk in the pudding so it thickens properly or the wrong amount, etc. From the point of view of treatment, exposure to and guidance in activities give the children more opportunities to achieve success. But at the same time it is also possible to observe how children react to this opportunity. Although it is perhaps hard to believe, some disturbed children find success hard to cope with. They may feel that people will expect more from them in the future—perhaps more than they feel able, or want, to give. Activities and children's responses to them are very revealing along these lines.

After expending considerable effort, Jimmy, an intelligent withdrawn child, completed a tile project. But before a surprised worker could stop him, he quickly and deliberately swept the work onto the floor, spoiling it. Through the worker's observation of Jimmy's reaction to his success, the child's therapist was able to probe with Jimmy the reasons for his being unable to accept it.

For other children failure is hard to accept. This is often brought out around game activities, in which they have difficulty in abiding by the rules.

Bud, a ten-year-old acting-out child on a treatment unit, could not tolerate the blow to his ego represented by losing in a game. If he was playing cards and losing, somehow he would manage to sweep everyone's cards off the table, making sure nobody else won either. If the group was playing a dice game, somehow his dice would be nudged so that he would get the number he needed to get ahead. If confronted by another child or a worker for cheating, he would have a tantrum. The workers' observations of Bud's behavior in these situations provided a means for both workers and other members of his treatment team to help him deal with the basic feelings behind his surface behavior.

In the course of participation in activities, praise or criticism is inevitably given. Although so much a part of normal children's and adults' daily lives, praise and criticism evoke varied reactions from disturbed children. To help the children with their feelings, staff have to be able to observe them in situations which elicit these feelings. Hard to believe as it is, some children have negative reactions to praise, wanting possibly to continue the unpleasant but easier role of not doing, nor having to do, anything praiseworthy.

Ken had just finished making a painting in an art session. A worker came by and told him what a nice painting it was. As soon as the worker had passed, Ken picked up a brush dripping with black paint and quickly scrubbed over his original painting.

Eleven-year-old Hank was interested in making models but needed some supportive guidance from workers to get the pieces in the right places. However, even the most positively phrased suggestion, such as, "Let's put this piece over there where the diagram has it marked," would be taken as direct criticism by this sensitive boy. But the very act of making models with Hank brought out reactions which it was important for all to be aware of and understand in planning his total treatment.

Activities provide workers also with the opportunity to gauge their children's reactions to structured and unstructured tasks. The structured ones, of course, are those which are highly defined —where the directions, procedures, and operations are more directed so that there are fewer alternative responses possible. Building an electric motor, for example, is a highly structured activity since each operation must be performed with precision in order for it to work. Clay, on the other hand, is an unstructured medium. There are many possible ways to handle it. In planning and carrying out a child's treatment program, it is important to be able to gauge how he reacts to tasks of varying degrees of structure.

Don, in an evaluation session, was given a lump of clay. Suddenly he seemed to freeze, looking at the clay as if it were something from Mars. Something in the characteristics of the clay had great significance for Don, reminding him of something that had frightened him deeply. Reports of this observation from the child care workers helped his therapist uncover important events in his past which were related to his reaction.

Sally would never attempt any but the most highly structured activity, such as numbered paintings or tile work. She would become paralyzed with anxiety when confronted by a plastic material such as finger paint. As with Don, exposure to the activities revealed important aspects of her personality.

Indeed, activities can provide important insights into the children's individual dynamics along various dimensions of behavior. They also provide a means to help children develop their interpersonal skills.

Having introduced the worker to the ways in which his initiative in activity program will bring therapeutic and managerial results, we can now turn to dealing with some of the more practical concerns in activity programming. How does one plan activities that will work with severely disturbed children? How does one get an activity started? What can one do to make it progress smoothly? The subsequent sections of this chapter will address themselves to these practical aspects of programming and others, offering guidelines and some specific activity suggestions for several types of participants under various circumstances.

Administration of Activities

Involved in the overall issue of executing an activity are factors related to the selection of the activity, preparation for the activity, and execution of the activity with the group.

Selection of Activities

When the worker starts to select an activity for his group of children, he needs to consider what specific and general goals he wishes to achieve through the activity. Ideally, he should choose something that will achieve treatment goals both for individual children and for the whole group. This is sometimes hard to arrange, but if the worker puts some thought into the reasons for the presentation of a particular activity at a specific time, he should be able to come up with something from which everyone can derive some benefit.

Activity analysis. One of the major aspects of making an activity selection is the worker's awareness of some of the elements of activities—their characteristics along various dimensions. For example, what exactly is involved in finger painting? What motions or operations are required? Can, or should, the children for whom the activity is being selected show an interest in it? How much competition, if any, is involved? Questions like these can be answered through the making of an "activity analysis." A term borrowed from the field of occupational therapy, it refers to the breaking down of an activity to see what its components are and how they can be matched to treatment goals. For example, three dimensions along which activities can be analyzed and which are relevant to treating disturbed children are body motions required, amount of competition and interaction involved, and degree of structure inherent in the activity.

With severely disturbed children, particularly highly withdrawn ones with poorly developed awareness of their bodies, selection of an activity along the lines of the physical motions involved can be most effective. Let us say that the worker is trying to pick an activity for a small group of withdrawn children, some of whom have deficiencies in perceptual functioning. For a group time with these children, the worker may wish to select something that will support development of these functions by requiring the children to use certain body motions. Even more specifically, he may feel that something that will help develop the concept of in and out, over and under is indicated. He then may consider what activities include these motions. As he thinks about arts and crafts, he may think of weaving, which of course requires in-out and/or over-under motions. Even if there are only paper and scissors on hand, he may be able to carry out the activity with the children by help-

ing them make woven paper mats. To illustrate further how activities can by analzyed according to the physical motions required,
table 1 represents an activity analysis of arts and crafts activities.

Table 1
ACTIVITY ANALYSIS

Motion	Basic Activity Form	Sample Activities
In and out, over and under with arm and hand	Weaving	Basketry Raffia Sewing Sewing cards Pot holders Rug-making Mat-making Cord-knotting
Right-left arm and hand coordination	Stringing	Stringing beads, macaroni, etc. Lacing (e.g., leather work) Sewing Chair-making
Circular	Stirring	Mixing plaster of Paris Mixing paint Mixing paper-mache Drilling
	Wrapping	Paper-mache strip application Raffia
Up and down, using arm strength and wrist grasp	Pounding	Clay work Hammering Metal craft Leather-tooling
Up and down, using open palm	Slapping	Clay work Paper-mache strip application Gluing Blot-painting
Controlled arm and hand suspension	Pouring	Paint preparation Mold-pouring

Motion	Basic Activity Form	Sample Activities
Back and forth arm extension and return	Painting	Painting with brush Spatter-painting
	Carpentry	Sawing Sanding Filing
	Pulling	Weaving rugs, mats, pot holders Lacing Cord-knotting
Hand closing and grasping with strength	Squeezing	Glue application Paper-mache strip application Clay work, other molding techniques
	Cutting	Paper sculpture, etc.
Precise arm-hand movement	Placing	Tile work Other mosaic-like crafts Popsicle-stick craft
Grasp and release	Dropping	Collages Decorating with glitter and similar materials

If the children have just been involved in a quiet activity, a worker may often feel that they should have a subsequent one which permits more physical motion. Here again he can look at the pool of available activities to see which might be most appropriate in terms of providing the physical outlet but also be relevant to the physical orientation of the children. For example, severely withdrawn children who prefer circular motion might be more responsive to circle games than to a game of basketball, which, indeed, they would not have the skills or conceptual understanding for anyway. To give another example, since severely disturbed, withdrawn children have many fears related to body intactness, they would not feel comfortable playing a swift game of dodge ball, whereas it might be just the thing to drain off energy in a group of older acting-out boys who are in a fairly cheerful mood.

Then, also, various activities require, or encourage, differing degrees of interaction and, in the case of games, competition among the children. This dimension is another one the worker may wish to analyze as he selects an activity. For example, in a group of children of mixed pathology (some acting-out verbal ones, some highly withdrawn ones), workers might wish to avoid team sports which the more withdrawn ones could probably not perform as well as the more active ones and which would probably only result in anger between the two types of children. To illustrate:

A worker in charge of a group of acting-out boys had just brought them back from a dog-eat-dog competition in softball with a group from another institution; his group had lost the game. All of the boys were glum, and there was some scapegoating of a few boys who had made errors which contributed toward the loss. After the boys had been back in their living space for a while relaxing, the worker knew, by the carping that was beginning to take place, that it was time to offer them something to do. The thought of a Monopoly game ran through his head; however, he knew that it was not going to be wise to involve them in anything else this day that would encourage a competitive type of interaction. What about work on their individual model kits? He decided against this too. With the pitch of frustration they were feeling, they might not tolerate the delicate, controlled work involved. He finally decided that he would get out his guitar for some group folk-singing—a passive, noncompetitive, nonfrustrating activity that would help rechannel the boys' negative feeling toward the few and would not pit them against one another.

Finally, the degree of structure inherent in an activity is another dimension that a worker can analyze as he plans his program. Chapter 7 describes this key term in reference to the degree of organization present in the total milieu. Its meaning is somewhat similar for specific activities, referring to the degree to which the materials and equipment define the task. In planning activities for different kinds of children, this is an important dimension to be taken into account. For example, a Monopoly game is more structured than a game of tag. There is really only one way to play the former, whereas the latter permits more individual latitude. As another example, building a model airplane is more structured than finger painting. The operations are precise and directed to make the plane; they can be quite random in finger painting. Making a bed, an activity requiring complex and precise movements, is more structured than wiping off a table. In working with disturbed children, it is often not simple to select an activity with the appropriate degree of structure, since the level of structure can have a direct effect on the type of response the worker receives to the activity.

A worker was assisting in a classroom for acting-out adolescent boys. One day she brought some modeling clay as part of her teaching materials. Much to her chagrin, when the boys received the clay, rather than beginning to shape objects with it, they began working pieces off and throwing them at one another. Finally, in a frenzy of glee, they began trying to see who could make pieces stick on the ceiling.

This activity was not appropriate for these boys. Although they were not, perhaps, capable of working on their own age level in school, they nonetheless knew that unstructured modelling clay was not a *school* type of material for boys of their age, and in a sense they reacted to it in the way in which it defined them.

A worker presented several withdrawn children with lumps of clay, with the expectation that the material would bring out true creative expression in the children. All the children did with it was to smell and finger it.

Again, for these particular children at their stage of development, this highly unstructured activity was not much more appropriate than a game of Monopoly. The children simply did not have the inner resources to deal with an activity at either extreme of the structure dimension. These illustrations are by no means intended to indicate that clay is not a suitable material for disturbed children (under appropriate circumstances it is, of course) but rather to show how the structure factor in activities can affect the children's responses. As a general rule of thumb, activities with a moderate degree of structure are often most effective with both acting-out and psychotic children, for the task indicates to some extent what must be done but the requirements are not so rigid that the children have neither the conceptual level nor the self-control to meet them.

The ability to analyze the various components of activities will aid the worker in the broader aspect of activity selection, which involves coordination of the activity with the rest of the children's program. This simply means that the activity taking place at any one time is appropriate in terms of what the children have done preceding the current activity, in terms of what they will be doing following it, and in terms of their current therapeutic needs. The term coordination also implies variation in type of activity; it is usually prudent to provide different kinds of activities during a day. This does not mean, however, that one activity cannot be related to another, since, in fact, some of the most effective activity programming is that in which the different types of activities have similar content. In checking with other departments workers may find out, for example, that children in school are studying plant growth. In conjunction with this subject, then, unit staff might plan nature walks or plant seeds as a unit project. When there is a program coordinator available, the broader coordination of activities, particularly across departments, would be his responsibility; however, workers still usually have many hours to plan for their group. This is where refined skills in activity selection and coordination make a great difference in the quality and effectiveness of what takes place.

Interest patterns of children.   It may seem obvious to say that selecting activities to relate to the expressed interests of the children is beneficial. However, with psychotic, severely disturbed children, whose primary interest might be spinning objects or some other repetitive activity, or even with more active, verbal children, whose emotional and intellectual functioning might not be adequate to every task, the picture becomes more complicated.

With the latter type of child, the challenge is to select activities that are appropriate and typical of his age, yet can be performed by the child. As was illustrated by the first anecdote about the clay, this kind of child is hair-trigger sensitive to being "put down" by being offered activities he feels are beneath him. Selection of an activity closely related to his interests often permits him to perform at a higher level.

An activity worker was trying to work with Johnny, an adolescent boy, to encourage him to develop more self-control and ability to take pleasure in manual activities. Although he ploddingly would do such things as cord-knotting, woodburning, and linoleum-block printing, the activities which really made him respond with more zest than anyone had ever observed were building an electric motor from a kit and making a model airplane. His investment and interest in the latter projects, closely related to the interests of normal boys of his age, allowed him to accept some of the extra frustrations which were inherent in them.

However, the most subtle application of the principle of relating activity choice to children's interest patterns is with severely disturbed children. With these children, so reluctant to engage in any activity other than their own bizarre choice, it is nonetheless possible to select activities that may appeal to them through relationship to their mode of symptomatic expression and, through the use of these activities, to encourage the children's participation in those which are more growth-producing. For example, many psychotic children respond to activities that appeal to basic senses, that is, to smell, touch, and hearing. Cooking activities, in particular, can be highly successful with this type of children since they usually are interested in food. As another example, psychotic children seem to respond to rhythm; thus activities which require rhythmic motion often evoke a positive response. Action songs, some forms of woodworking, and simple household tasks are several which contain this appealing rhythmic component. This pattern of behavior in a child is different from that in many children who, in order to feel less self-conscious when talking to adults, are helped by having some small object to twiddle in their fingers.

While most children need special help in becoming effective participants in activities, there are some children who almost need the opposite—to be focussed away from activities. These are children who too readily involve themselves with some kind of activity, which they may carry out as a way to avoid grappling with their feelings and relating to other people, and workers should be alert to spot them. This type of child, who may *always* have his nose in a book or his shoulders hunched over a craft or game, might be easy to manage but may also be missing out on important interpersonal experiences. The child who intrusively and inevitably changes the subject by saying, "Let's play cards" or, "I'm going to make my next lanyard red and blue" when workers are trying to discuss behavior or feelings with him may be one of these. If a worker feels that a child in his group is using activities in this way, he should probably describe the child's behavior to the supervisor or therapist and gain suggestions on how to handle it.

Some children, in particular acting-out ones, may be very interested in an activity, but only in one, seeming to be fixated on one type of craft or game to the exclusion of anything else. This type of child, having achieved competence in this one area, is often afraid to try anything else. Here it is the task of workers to select activities that are so appealing—as well as being within the child's ability range—that the child can hardly resist trying them or to select another activity which has elements similar to those of the favored activity.

Group characteristics. In selecting an activity, the worker needs to consider various group factors, both among the children and among the staff. First of all, the available staff will help determine what activities are selected. If a worker is on duty by himself, he may not want to involve a group of acting-out children in wood carving, which he cannot adequately supervise from the point of view either of safety or of craftsmanship. He might instead encourage the children to play active games of medium structure that do not require close supervision. If the group is comprised of withdrawn children, this again would be the time when the worker might not attempt an activity in which each child would need individual guidance. Rather, he might try a group activity in which participation would be more passive, such as listening to records. If there are several workers on duty at a particular time, a more complex activity can be selected. Several groups of children can work on different aspects of it, and one worker can be assigned to each group. For example, in making a group collage, one subgroup of children can mix paint; another can cut up scraps; another can be gluing them on the paper as they are ready.

The size of the children's group and the type of children in it will also play a part in determining the selection of activities. Activities for large groups must by necessity be less highly structured and need less specific guidance for their success than those for smaller groups. For a group of psychotic children the activities selected would probably not require the ability to conceptualize and verbalize that might be required in activities that would be suitable for older acting-out children. For example, older active children often enjoy card and table games when they are not upset. Psychotic children have, for the most part, little ability to participate in them; games for them must be simple and based more on physical activity.

The children's ability to make their own choices and their interest in doing so are naturally key factors in the selection of activities. Psychotic children may need much direction from the staff in making choices, but children who are less disturbed may well have, and should be encouraged to express, their own ideas. The worker can then help put these suggestions into effect if in his clinical judgment they are appropriate. Participation in the decision-making process is actually an important element of the children's treatment. The role of the worker is to provide necessary guidelines and support, being constantly on the lookout for cues as to when the children are ready for more and more active participation in their own programming. When a group of disturbed children is selecting its activities, the worker should be alert for such problems as the most verbal child who always states his choice in such a way that he drowns out the more reticent ones who may also have ideas and the child whose choice of activity is always deeply related to his disturbance so that the activity would not really be beneficial to the group. Many disturbed children have little previous experience upon which to base a choice of a constructive activity, but as the worker uses his knowledge and skills to enrich the children's activity diet, he will see that they will be developing more and more background upon which to make their own choices and will begin to be able to do so in a healthy fashion.

There are, of course, other group factors which would influence a worker's selection of an activity. It is not necessary to elaborate upon all of them but simply to point out to the worker that an important element to consider when planning program is the characteristics of the group.

This section on the selection of an activity may give the worker the impression that the process is a complicated one. However, once a worker is oriented to and has had some experience in carrying out activities with disturbed children, he sees that he is often able to make a fairly quick and adequate judgment as to what is appropriate at a certain time for a particular group. When involved with a group of children, one would hardly expect a worker to sit down and make a complicated activity analysis—he would not have any energy left to carry out the activity with the children. Rather, the purpose of describing in detail the elements of the selection process is to provide the worker with a background that he can use to guide his on-the-spot decisions more effectively.

Preparation for Activities

Once a worker has selected an activity, he must usually make preparations in order to carry it out with the children, and preparation can have a direct effect on the success and outcome of the activity. As with the selection process, we would again emphasize that the worker need not agonize over every detail to the extent that he is too exhausted to carry out the activity or feels that nothing can be done on a spur-of-the-moment basis. Frequently a worker must pull an activity out of nowhere to meet an on-the-spot need for some kind of program. It is useful, however, to point out some aspects of activities which, if given some thought ahead of time, help everything go along well. The following examples may illustrate:

Three workers in an evening woodshop program did a wonderful job of helping the children make storage boxes for their treasures. One evening two of the workers were sick, leaving one worker responsible for the group. This worker thought that perhaps he would have the boys paint their boxes that night. Since he was the only one on duty, he did not have a chance to go into the shop ahead of the boys (he would have had to be away from the group) to check things first: to make sure that all boxes were ready for painting, that the paint was ready, that sufficient rags and turpentine for cleanup were on hand. The result was chaos. The boys blew into the room. The worker wished that he were an octopus as he tried to meet simultaneously demands from "Help me finish this so I can paint like the others are" to "Open this – – – can of paint." He had to keep one boy from snatching the brush from another's hand and dunking it into a can of paint of a different color; he had to help the boys learn the appropriate way of applying enamel paint rather than just "slopping" it on. To complicate matters further, the worker could not find the turpentine to clean up mistakes on the boxes and paint-covered hands, resulting in the paint's getting on some good furniture outside the activity room. The boys themselves were not pleased with the results of the painting and for the first time were angry and disappointed with their boxes.

Careful activity selection and preparation could have prevented this disaster from taking place. Another incident shows how preparation contributed to some of the joys of child care work:

Jane and Barb, two child care workers, were on duty with a group of school-age children to whom they were interested in introducing their shared interest, astronomy. On a clear day (in anticipation of a clear night) each worker brought in her telescope, a few astronomy books, and a few star-finder charts to help locate the constellations. After dinner, as the group returned to their unit from the dining room, the two workers talked about how they were going to set up and conduct the activity. They decided, first of all, that Jane would set up the telescopes in the back activity room, which had a good outlook to the sky, just before it got dark, while Barb would keep the group busy. They knew that the excitement of watching and waiting while the workers set up the telescopes in front of them would be too much for the children. Jane would also lay out the star finders in two different places and select a few easy-to-find constellations to show the group. Then, before bringing the children into the activity room, the workers would divide them into two groups, one for each telescope, and explain what the procedures would be before they actually entered the room, with emphasis on the fact that they would need to take turns with the telescopes. The activity proceeded in a pleasant and productive fashion. The children in each group, sharing among themselves a telescope and a star finder, found they did not have to wait long and could wait patiently since they knew what to expect. Each worker kept her eye on the children in her subgroup and made sure that none was distressed or unoccupied; the group division made this possible.

Using this anecdote as an example, we can spell out what is involved in preparing to carry out an activity.

Selection of a physical setting. Once an activity is planned, the worker should plan to conduct it in an area that is appropriate both for the type of children who will be involved and for the activity. For example, a painting activity such as described in the first anecdote would not be carried out in the living area of the unit. The activity would have had to be limited so closely that it would have been sabotaged from the start. A group of children would not be encouraged to play dodge ball in a tiny TV room— there would not be much freedom of activity for the children. In both anecdotes the workers gave consideration to picking an area which would support the purpose of the activity.

Arrangement of materials and equipment. Making sure that all the necessary materials were available, accessible, and in good working order contributed toward the success of the telescope activity. As a further example, a model-building session in which all glue bottles are easily flowing will be more successful than one in which they are stuck and everyone has to wait while they are opened. In arranging the materials for an activity ahead of time, some workers find it wise to keep out of the children's reach any items they do not want to be used immediately or without super-vision. For example, in tooling and lacing leather the children do not need the awl for punching holes until the tooling is finished and the holes are marked. Only then might the awl be brought out so that there would be little leeway for it to be misused. Although it is judicious to keep equipment that needs to be closely supervised out of sight until it is time to use it, it often helps to stimulate children's interest in the activity if some of the materials that are to be used are in view.

Planned staff assignments. Both anecdotes illustrate how suc-cess with activities is enhanced by planning what the roles of the available staff members will be. As already stated, some activities cannot be carried out with one or two staff members and should be postponed until a time when more help is available. These are usually activities which have some element of danger if not closely supervised (i.e., woodburning, swimming, cooking), are so com-plex that the children need extra help and support (i.e., model-building, learning a new table game), or involve considerable waiting and taking of turns (i.e., the telescope-viewing, cooking when there is only one bowl, relay races). Looser activities such as record playing, tumbling, simple card games, reading, storytelling, crayoning are more suitable for times when staff is short.

When the group of children is large, it is often helpful, as was suggested in chapter 7, to subdivide them into smaller groups, each under a worker. This helps both workers and children to direct their responses and makes for a smoother activity. Some-times staff find that it helps to assume different functions in car-rying out an activity: "While you're helping the children mix up the cake, I'll get the frosting ingredients out"; "When the young-sters are tired of string painting, I'll get a group to help clean up if you want to start some of the others with their showers."

Breaking down the act of preparing for an activity into speci-fic processes may make the job sound tedious, but this is not the case in real life. Workers find that with experience they automati-cally begin to think of these details, and the little extra effort required to carry them out results in their own enjoyment of successful joint experiences with their group.

Techniques for Effective Participation

It is helpful if, when the workers are ready to begin an activity with their group, they have knowledge of ways to handle the children while the activity is going on, so that the children get as much exposure to the activity as possible and so that it is sucessful. Following are some of the approaches which child care workers have found helpful in the ongoing direction of an activity:

Positive expectation. With normal children one automatically expects that they will want to participate in activities. With disturbed children, however, one may be so puzzled and put off by their bizarre behavior and surface resistance that he gets the idea that the children cannot really do much and that not much should be expected of them by way of participation in various activities. Indeed, if approached with an attitude of "Well, we really don't feel you are going to go along with us on this," the children probably will not. Instead, the staff should approach the children with positive expectation. They simply present and conduct the activity in a way that shows the children that the staff are convinced of their willingness and ability to perform and participate—are convinced that, of course, they will join in when asked. This concept may sound nebulous, but actually it is related to the accepted premise in work with psychotic children that staff should be direct and explicit in their approach, helping to reduce the children's confusion by structuring the situation for them.

Examples can demonstrate how positive expectation helps the child. Often the results of the staff's positive approach, even if only indirectly conveyed to the children, are seen when the children are taken on an outing away from their living unit. On return from such a trip, workers sometimes comment on how well the children behaved when out, even if they are already slipping back into symptomatic actions. Perhaps one reason for this phenomenon is the message that the children get: "You are out in public now, and we know you can—and must—act as you should."

An activity worker approached Carol, a school-age child, about coming to her craft session on an afternoon when she had apparently been quite upset, wandering around aimlessly, making bizarre noises, and seeming to be quite inaccessible. Carol attempted to avoid the worker and squirmed away when her hand was taken. The worker was not put off and kept talking to Carol, telling her that she wanted her to come and knew she could "make it." Carol suddenly relaxed, came readily, and had a productive session. The expectation that she could and would participate led to success.

A psychotic boy who at times could perform with ease would also have periodic outbursts in which he would lose control, throwing whatever he was working on across the room. When workers began to appeal to his dignity by saying, "Come on, control yourself; I *know* you can do it!" conveying to him that they were convinced that he could manage his feelings better, he would usually settle down and continue what he was doing.

Utilization of specific symptomatic patterns. The idea of building activities around specific behavioral characteristics of the children to gain their initial response was cited in the section on the selection of activities, but this principle is so important that it can again be discussed as a means to engage certain children's participation in ongoing activities. It is amazing how many symptomatic actions of disturbed children can be employed in the service of ego-building, constructive activities. Disturbed motility patterns, such as preference for circular motion in psychotic children, compulsiveness (the tendency to repeat the same act over and over or to impose a rigid arrangement or order on things), and aggression, all can be channelled into programmed activities. The following examples illustrate:

In the craft area of a treatment center for psychotic children, it was observed that some of the most withdrawn children had an almost automatic tendency to stir anything placed in front of them. This appeared to be an action that did not have to be taught and of course seemed related to their characteristic preference for circular motion. Even in the very early stages of the craft program on this unit, when the children were resistant and inaccessible, all one had to do to gain their participation was to place a dish of paint, plaster, paper-mache, etc., in front of them, and, presto, with no direction at all, they would take the stirring stick and stir competently. This served to incorporate the contributions of these withdrawn children into several constructive group craft projects in which more adequate children performed other operations.

Jane showed pronounced compulsiveness as well as excellent manual dexterity and coordination; in the playroom she was frequently observed to move objects just the tinest bit to fit some need she had for rigid order. In crafts, which she initially tended to resist, her participation was gained through projects which could utilize her need for objects to be placed in a certain orderly way, such as making things with tiles and popsicle sticks. She turned out to be an expert at using these materials. She would carefully put glue on sticks and tiles and place them just right, thereby constructing a number of meaningful objects which brought her praise and also widened her range of interests.

The idea of using substitute activities to rechannel the aggression present in so many children may be one of the "oldest saws" in child care work, but it nonetheless seems to be true that angry feelings can be put into the service of ongoing participation in a related activity.

Joe, for example, was a child who frequently bit when anxious or angry. He enjoyed learning how to saw during activity periods and actually seemed to be able to use this activity rather than to use his teeth to bite.

One may feel that simply utilizing symptomatic characteristics in activities does not really serve as a basis for helping the child grow and change. Let us clarify the point. When a child is behaving symptomatically on his own, he is probably not exposing himself to new patterns of stimulation or to social interaction. When he does this in the context of an activity, however, inevitably he is having contact with different kinds of media and experiences and with those directing the activity who react to what he does. The symptomatic patterns utilized help bring the child into this wider area of experiences.

Individual help and support for maintenance of appropriate behavior. Individual help and support consist of the staff members' taking a directive role with the child to help him maintain himself in an activity. The worker accepts the child at his own level but gives him as much support and encouragement as necessary to keep him effectively involved—the staff member being, in a sense, a "co-ego." For some children this support may involve their being led through the whole activity by the worker, but the effort is worthwhile since the children are constantly being made aware of themselves as the adult continues to focus them on the task at hand. An example of this technique is given by Cumming and Cumming, who describe a recreational therapist who placed regressed schizophrenics in position to play a simple game of ball and encouraged them to participate, gradually making the game more complex.[1] This technique of acting as a co-ego has been performed many times with severely disturbed children in one treatment center. When these children first began attending a newly established craft program, it was necessary for workers to provide much support. The children would, unless limited by the adults, quickly fall into their characteristic mannerisms—twirling objects, playing with string, flapping fingers, etc. However, when the adult gently but firmly intruded, it was easy to direct each child back to the activity at hand. This was done by gently turning the child's head back toward the activity or replacing the object he might be twirling with another and showing him how to use it appropriately.

Jon, age eight, would paint a few strokes correctly or would squeeze glue a few times. Then he might begin to twirl either object around. To redirect this activity, it was only necessary to gently stop his hands, place the object in an appropriate position, and then start him off again using it correctly.

This particular approach is somewhat more relevant to working

1. John Cumming and Elaine Cumming, *Ego and Milieu: Theory and Practice of Environmental Therapy* (New York, 1962), p. 151.

with psychotic children than with acting-out verbal children, although the latter also need a special kind of guidance and support from workers as they encounter the inevitable frustrations inherent in activities. The reader may be saying at this point, "Well, this is fine but we never have enough staff to give each child this type of attention." This statement could well be true, and true most of the time. But nonetheless there are times when a worker can focus on an entire group and still move around giving a number of children individual support periodically. In many settings these days, also, there are students and volunteers available to assist workers in carrying out activities, and often a valuable role for them to assume is that of providing special support for certain children while the regular worker directs an ongoing activity.

Introduction of a new object into the environment. A technique for engaging severely disturbed children in activities and spearheading their continued involvement is to introduce into their program something completely novel—a new toy, a new craft material, or an activity involving a change of routine. It has been observed in some treatment centers that although many disturbed children resist substantial changes in their environment, they gravitate toward a new plaything that has just been introduced. They not only show appropriate curiosity but also show more direct interest in it than is characteristic of their day-to-day behavior toward objects. Thus occasional introduction of a completely new object or material can be a useful program technique, in that it often results in more purposeful and directed behavior from the children. This would seem to be an especially useful strategy for times when the children are not involved in a formally structured activity with direct instruction from adults, since it would give them "booster stimulation" to apply learnings from more structured situations in unstructured ones, to learn to play appropriately, and to become interested in the physical world.

At one treatment center the children's playroom was fairly small, containing standard children's play equipment such as blocks and a playhouse. One day, during a transitional period (while the children were waiting for school to begin), they were milling around aimlessly until a large, yellow, brand-new ball was introduced. The effect of this ball on the children, particularly the sicker ones, was impressive. Many went directly over to it and began exploring and playing with it. Larry, a disturbed verbal child not given to making positive statements, said, "I like it," voluntarily. Janet, a girl who spent most of her free time in repetitive play with small objects, went over to the ball and without direction or encouragement patted and bounced it.

In another treatment center, one afternoon a new wooden train with wheels on it, which could be ridden by the children, was brought into the playroom. Jane left her customary solitary bizarre preoccupations, went directly to the train, climbed on it, and rode around pushing appropriately with her feet.

Alternation of structured with unstructured activities. The success of any given activity can depend in part on what the children were doing before the activity began. Many workers find that periods of structured, directed activities are more successful when they are alternated with periods of less structured activity. If children have been in a loose situation for a while, they are more able to accept—or even want—direct guidance and intervention in their activity.

It is important to point out that the unstructured time which we are describing as being so important in the overall scheme of programming does not mean that there should be nothing available for the children to do. Rather this would be more of a time of free choice of activity by the children from a variety of safe, developmentally oriented materials. The crucial function of free play in the lives of children has been stressed in chapter 5; it is during these periods of less structure and direction that children can be provided this essential experience. The job of the staff is to serve more as background observers and facilitators, rather than as active directors of the activity. They may see that appropriate materials are available—construction toys such as Lego and Lincoln Logs; clay; crayons, scissors, paint, paper; dolls,

trucks, and other playthings which stimulate the children's imagi-
nations; games; softballs and tossing objects such as a frisbee;
wheel and skill toys such as scooters, bicycles, and roller skates,
to name just a few. A more detailed list of appropriate free-play
materials is found in the Appendix to this chapter.

These materials can be offered for free play with minimal staff
involvement in direct organization or used for specific activity
purposes in which the staff plays a stronger directive part. We
should reiterate that periods of free play are not times when the
staff members quickly say, "It will be free-play time now" and
withdraw from the group completely. Rather, staff are available
to children in the same way they make the materials available;
they intervene when necessary to protect rights and safety and
occasionally perhaps to give a child sufficient boosts to get started
playing productively, and they respond when approached by the
children. The periods of free activity give the children the opportunity to try to apply skills learned in regular activities, prevent
too much intrusion by adults which might increase the children's
negativism, provide the staff the opportunity to observe the children's level of functioning as a measure of their ability to consolidate gains made in other areas, and, most importantly, give the
children the opportunity to mobilize their forces before entering
a new activity. An additional benefit from alternation of structured and less structured activities is that the children's awareness
of the difference in quality in the environment aids their perception of time and space by changing in a systematic way the pattern of stimulation they receive. The relevance of delineating
time and space in the service of providing a therapeutic milieu
is pointed out in chapter 7.

Emphasis on the finished product.   The way in which activities
are conducted often depends on what the worker's goals are in
terms of finished products. While finished products are usually
associated with arts and crafts, there are other activities too in
which a state of completion can be reached, such as cooking,
clean-up tasks, and some games. In conducting activities, then,
workers need to understand when a finished product or com-

pleted activity is relevant to the treatment goals and development of the child or group, and to what degree this should be emphasized in the ongoing directing of the activity.

Beginning workers sometimes feel either that the end effort of an activity is of no importance (they say, "It doesn't really matter how it turns out") or that there must be, in the culmination of the child's efforts, a fine-looking piece of work, no matter how much adult structuring and directing has been involved. By examining some aspects of programming related to the finished product, we can see on what basis a worker might develop a decision on this for a given child.

First of all, part of the stress that might or might not be placed on the finished product will be determined by the nature of the project or activity itself. Materials lending themselves to expressive activity such as painting and collage work may, with disturbed children, require guidance and support for appropriate use, but may not require focus on the finished product for the children to enjoy and benefit from the activity. Here, indeed, the stress is on the process more than the product. When people evaluate products of expressive activities, too, they are more able to accept—or should be—say, a mélange of color on a piece of paper which does not look like anything than a model airplane with one wing missing, one on crooked, and gobs of extra glue smeared all over it.

A worker was interested in what would happen if the children tried out something she had just heard about—painting to music. Since the children were especially responsive to music, she thought it might be a worthwhile and enjoyable activity. The children were more manageable and concentrated longer during the project than usual, and when they were finished, all the workers were pleased. Yet no child had produced a painting of "something." In looking at the papers, one could see simply a random array of strokes. In this activity the gains were made in the doing, and the final product simply did not matter.

More structured materials, on the other hand, imply more emphasis on what the final result looks like. Here is where the worker must strike a balance between the way in which he guides a child in an activity (what performance level he encourages and expects) and the child's need to have his finished product look good. For example, a very disturbed, withdrawn, nonverbal child might, under great pressure and direction, be able to produce a passable model airplane from a simple kit but would gain no sense of having made the achievement on his own. He might, however, with simple guidance, be able to perform the motions necessary to make a box out of popsicle sticks or a mosaic-tile hot plate, to the extent that the final result would look reasonably good and yet the child could feel that it came about largely by his own efforts.

With these kinds of materials, in most instances, it is actually important that the worker at least guide the child sufficiently so that, within flexible limits, the end product is presentable. Probably the most disturbed child is aware of his own disorganization; seeing it mirrored in a product that directly reflects his own chaos is not always healthy for his self-esteem. Furthermore, poor results are often reflected back by other children, who may make such comments as, "Boy, that mess looks like John."

With younger children, with highly withdrawn children, and particularly with those who have previously shown little evidence of concrete achievement, productions have special meaning to parents, who see them as tangible evidence of progress. Sometimes, a child's beginning accomplishments, made as the result of careful activity selection and guidance by his child care worker, contribute toward giving the child a more positive image in his parents' eyes.

A child care worker brought Tim, a very withdrawn child, to saw in the woodwork shop. Using the simple back-and-forth motion to saw and the up-and-down motion to hammer, Tim was able, as a result of the worker's showing him where to saw and hammer, to make a small wooden box which he then painted and took home on a weekend visit. Later the social worker reported that the parents had told her that they were amazed. They had never realized that Tim could do anything like this. Experiences like this gradually helped the parents change their image of Tim as a child who would be unable to learn.

Older, more reality-oriented, and acting-out verbal children have other kinds of special needs for adequately finished products. Here there is more than the possible reflection of their competence and status at stake; there is also the idea that the product may be of specific use to them. It is in some ways more difficult to work with acting-out children in activities; their impulsiveness and lack of frustration tolerance show in their performance; they are aware, more than the frankly psychotic child, of the effect of their pathology on their performance. It is a delicate balance for the worker to achieve: to guide their activities so that the results are acceptable to them but not to overdirect them to an extent that they cannot tolerate. The importance of presentable work to older verbal children is illustrated by the following example:

Through a gradual process of increasing expectation for good quality work, a worker in a state hospital with acting-out preadolescent boys found that these boys were making handsome projects with wood that to a large degree reflected their own effort; she was supplying mostly background guidance and suggestions. Pleased with this achievement of her group, the worker was disconcerted to hear that the boys, rather than keeping their products for themselves, were selling them to unit attendants. She felt that since the boys had put so much effort into their work, they should keep the results for themselves. A supervisor, however, was able to clarify her thinking: the success in workmanship that the boys had achieved could bring them tangible rewards. They were experiencing a basic tenet of our society—that a good job can command respect and compensation in the form of money. For these children, previously accustomed to the experience of failure, this achievement was probably their first experience with society's rewards for success.

A project leading to a finished product which is either highly appropriate in terms of age-level interest value or related to an expressed interest of a child can lead him to perform in a more adequate fashion than he may previously have done simply because he truly wants the finished product.

A worker was having an activity session with an adolescent boy who had had little of that experience with making things which is customary in the development of normal children. Although he made some effort on projects that adults might like, such as ashtrays, he nonetheless did not seem to be giving his all to the work nor seem very pleased when he finished something. The worker obtained for him a kit from which an electric buzzer system could be built. The change in his approach was remarkable. Although he could barely read, he would pore over the instructions, trying to follow them step by step. If he made a mistake or encountered a difficult part, he stuck with it until he had mastered it. When the buzzer was finally finished, he was eager to take it back to his living area to show to the other boys. Here the special meaning of a finished product to a child had a positive effect on the process involved in finishing it.

In this discussion we have shed some light on the issue of finished products, showing how they are meaningful to certain children and under what circumstances this is so. Dealing effectively with this dimension of activity programming helps the child care worker make each activity as meaningful and profitable to the child as possible.

Conclusion

The Appendix to this chapter discusses briefly some major activity areas to give the worker who is planning the program for his group some general ideas of the many possibilities open to him. It will be his task to adapt each activity to the particular circumstances under which he is working and the particular needs of his group. The guidelines in this chapter should make this job a challenging but fulfilling one, as the worker begins to see the positive effects his efforts have on his charges' behavior, not only in the activity itself but in all of the children's experiences.

This chapter has provided a survey of some of the reasons for including programmed activities in the treatment of disturbed children and has pointed out the important function of the child care worker in this area, which has been too often neglected, both in the lives of the children and in the orientation of the worker. Activity programming, especially with severely disturbed children, is a challenging enterprise, requiring both a theoretical understanding of children's developmental needs and the more practical knowledge of which activities to pick to meet these needs and how to carry them out within the context of agency structure. For the worker who makes a wholehearted attempt to meet this challenge, however, there are rewards: the first of these may be the worker's knowledge that he has contributed not simply to a segmented part of a child's life but rather to his total development as a happy and productive individual. Secondly, he may, through the route of programming for the children, find a new interest or hobby for himself as well as build new relationships which will contribute to his own development as a person and to increased satisfaction as a professional child care worker.

Appendix to Chapter 12

Introduction

So that the child care worker can continue to develop in the area of putting theory into practice in activity programming, the following supplementary sections are presented:

1. Suggested Activity Areas
2. Bibliography of Activity Resources
3. Suggested Play Materials
4. Sources of Play Supplies and Equipment

It should be established at the outset that none of these sections is intended to be a comprehensive cookbook approach to carrying out activities. There are many other activity areas and specific activities than are named in the various sections. The role of this Appendix is simply to introduce the worker to some concrete sources that will help him begin his own search for ideas and materials with which to plan and implement activities for the children in his care. Activities are listed without particular categorization in terms of age and type of child or safety, developmental, therapeutic, and managemental factors. The worker must make his choices from the pool of possibilities and adapt them to his particular situation.

Suggested Activity Areas

The major purpose of Part IV has been to lay down a philosophy of, and guidelines for, activity programming for disturbed children so that the worker will have a background for adapting any type of activity to the particular needs and circumstances of his group. Our goal in the chapter was not to offer a cookbook of activity ideas: there are many other books available with specific directions for carrying out different activities for children, and, as we also stated previously, the worker, if he looks back to his own childhood, can undoubtedly recall many enjoyable activities in which he himself participated, and his co-workers will contribute similar ideas. With these resources on tap, the worker should have enough basic knowledge to be able to perform his specialized task of planning activities for a disturbed group. There are some activity areas, however, which are particularly suited for execution with disturbed children. This section describes briefly some of these activity areas and lists some specific activities within them, in the hope that they will stimulate the worker to continue a search for appropriate and meaningful activities for his group.

Arts and Crafts

Seemingly the largest activity area, arts and crafts can provide the backbone for any activity program. The possibilities for interesting and meaningful activities within this category are tremendous. There are several reasons for this: almost any kind of scrap or "everyday" material can be employed in the service of arts and crafts; needs for specialized equipment *can* be minimal. The same activity may appeal to and be within the ability level of a large variety of children. Arts and crafts range in degree of structure from the unstructured (e.g., plastic media such as paint) to the highly structured (e.g., weaving). They may be presented to encourage interaction (e.g., group projects) and even competition or to promote individual activity. A complete range of physical movements of the upper body can be tapped through arts and crafts activities.

Collage-making from
  Cloth scraps
  Cut straws
  Dried cereals and vegetables
  Macaroni and alphabet
    noodles
  Torn paper
Crayoning
  Crayon and watercolor
    drawings
  Crayon etchings
  Crayon rubbings
  Feather-crayon drawings
Hammering
  Leather-tooling
  Metal work (pounded
    ashtrays, etc.)
Lacing and stitching
  Embroidery
  Punched-leather lacing
    projects
  Sewing
  Sewing cards
Modelling
  Paper-mache (self-molded or
    using preconstructed base)
  Plaster of Paris (with molds)
Object-arranging
  Popsicle stick and tongue
    depressor projects
  Tile work
Painting
  Blow-painting with straws
  Ink-blot painting

Object-printing (carrot,
  potato)
Painting by the numbers
Painting on egg-carton
  liners
Spatter-painting
Sponge-painting
String-painting
Paper-folding and cutting
  Airplanes
  Chains
  Lanterns
  Origami
  Snowflakes
  Woven mats
Plastic media
  Clay
  Easel paints
  Finger paints
  Play dough
Weaving
  Basketry
  Cord-knotting
  Indian beads
  Lanyards
  Pot holders
  Raffia
  Rake-knitting
  Spool-knitting
Woodworking
  Boats
  Boxes
  Cars
  Scrapbooks
  Shelves

Sports and Games

Another area in which there is a wide variety of possible activities is sports and games. As with arts and crafts, some can be initiated with little if any special equipment; others require more props. Games often lack the wide appeal that crafts have to a large number of children. Those which are within the range of ability for severely withdrawn children (e.g., circle games) may not appeal to verbal, acting-out children, and conversely many sports and games enjoyed by verbal children are not within the range of understanding of most psychotic children. The greatest variety of physical movements is tapped by games and sports. Although there is the possibility for solitary play or practice on individual skills within the category of sports and games, most encourage interaction and, of course, some promote competition. While the degree of structure in sports and games varies, there seems to be some structure in all.

Active games, with equipment
  Hopscotch
  Jump rope
  Shuffleboard
  Tug-of-War
Active games, without
    equipment
  Giant Steps
  Hide-and-Seek
  Red Rover
  Sardines
  Simon Says
  Statues
  Stoop Tag
  Tag
Ball and bag games
  Beanbag games
  Bowling
  Call Ball

Dodge ball
  Monkey in the Middle
Circle games
  Cat and Rat
  Drop the Handkerchief
  Farmer in the Dell
  Musical Chairs
  Numbers Change
  Pass the Button (Shoe, etc.)
  Ring-Around-the-Rosy
Relay races
  Follow Through
  Over-Under
  Sack race
  Wheelbarrow
Small-group skill games
  Blockhead
  Jacks
  Pickup sticks

Wire puzzles	Table games, board
Sports, outdoor, individual	Bingo
Cycling	Checkers
Hiking	Chess
Playground equipment,	Chinese Checkers
swings, slide, etc.	Clue
Roller-skating	Monopoly
Swimming	Parcheesi
Sports, outdoor, team	Table games, card
Baseball	Bridge
Basketball	Canasta
Football	Casino
Handball	Discard
Softball	Hearts
Tennis	Old Maid
Sports, possible indoor	Slapjack
Frisbee	Solitaire
Ringtoss	Table games, paper and pencil
Roller-skating	Dots and Lines
Tumbling	Ships
	Tictactoe

Cooking

It may be surprising to see cooking proposed as a legitimate part of a children's activity program. Its therapeutic possibilities are so high that it would seem that it deserves consideration as an activity in its own right. Although, of course, there are some requirements for materials and equipment so that basic cooking activities can be performed, these can be quite simple, particularly for foods that do not have to be heated. Cooking involves a variety of physical movements and varying degrees of structure; the interaction-competition factor should be given particular consideration in making an activity analysis of a cooking project. Most cooking activities involve a group, with different individuals performing different functions. Since interest in food runs high in disturbed children, competition can arise for those jobs which get one closest to the food. With planning, however, workers can set up the activity either to promote or to discourage various kinds of interaction.

Heated foods
  Baked goods
  Hot chocolate
  Jello
  Popcorn
  Pudding
  Roasted marshmallows

Nonheated foods
  Cake, cookie decorations
  Crackers and spreads
  Drink mixes (Kool-Aid, chocolate)
  Frosting mixes
  Instant puddings
  Sandwiches

Household Tasks

Like cooking, household tasks are not usually considered a component of a formal activity program. However, these also have many therapeutic possibilities when used appropriately and are similar in many ways to other activities. The worker's efforts to allow and encourage the children to participate in the care of their surroundings permit valuable learning to take place and a special sense of pride to develop. Household tasks offer a range both of structure and of the physical movements required and can be either solitary or group endeavors. With children who can handle it, competition can be a motivating factor in performing household tasks. Psychotic children can perform many simple household tasks.

Complex tasks
  Emptying wastebaskets
  Folding clothes
  Hanging up clothes
  Making beds
  Putting away complex games
  Setting tables
  Sweeping and using dustpan

Simple tasks
  Mopping
  Moving furniture
  Picking up
  Putting objects in boxes, drawers, or shelves
  Throwing laundry in hamper
  Throwing trash in wastebaskets
  Wiping tables

Music

Like arts and crafts, music can be a mainstay on a unit of disturbed children. Musical activities have great appeal to disturbed children; although most do not require special ability for the workers to carry them out, they usually require some kind of special equipment, depending on the type of activity being planned. A wide range of bodily movements can be encouraged through various types of musical activities; the range in level of structure is great, going all the way from simple motions made to rhythms to the complex behavior required to play an instrument. Musical activities can promote either interaction, as in group singing, or solitude, as when individuals listen to a musical program.

Eurythmics

Group singing (rounds, action songs)

Individual performance on instrument

Musical games (Musical Chairs, etc.)

Record-playing

Rhythm band (with either commercial or homemade instruments)

Special Events

Special events play an important part in the treatment of disturbed children. As was emphasized in chapter 7, they can be invaluable in bringing staff and children together to work for a common goal and thus providing a means for much positive interaction. The criteria for planning and carrying out a special event are somewhat different from those for the more basic activities described previously, since preparation may take place over a long period of time and involve many individual activities which contribute to the final event. In a sense, a special event is a synthesis of several individual activity areas. For example, at a unit open house one might see the results of the children's activities in crafts, cooking, household tasks, and, if a performance is given, music.

Hunts
  Scavenger
  Treasure
Parties
  Birthday
  Farewell
  Holiday
  Open house
  Welcome
Performances
  Art show
  Plays
  Skits

Songs
Tumbling
Trips
  Airport
  Amusement park
  Factory
  Farm
  Flower show
  Outdoor concert
  Skating rink
  Sports event
  Zoo

Bibliography of Activity Resources

This list of books containing activity ideas is simply a brief selection from the tremendous body of literature describing activity areas and techniques. The literature cited here is primarily geared toward normal children within a wide age range; as we mentioned previously, the worker needs to choose and adapt a particular activity to his own circumstances.

It will be noted that a number of the books seem to be directed toward younger children. This should not deter the worker, however. Many of these activities are actually quite suited in content for disturbed children and for older children. Many of them are also suitable as sources for transitional activities, which are those brief time fillers which a worker has on tap to make moments of waiting between one part of the day's schedule and another enjoyable and even constructive, rather than fraught with restless behavior from the children and unpleasant controls from the workers.

Many of the listed books are available in paperback, thereby making them more accessible. Examination of the bibliographies in many of the books will provide the worker with further leads on sources of activity ideas and techniques.

Boston Children's Medical Center and Gregg, Elizabeth M. *What to Do When There's Nothing to Do*. New York: Dell, 1968. Paperback.

Burnett, Dorothy Kirk. *Your Preschool Child: Making the Most of the Years From 2 to 7*. New York: MacFadden Bartell, 1963. Paperback.

Comstock, N., ed. *McCall's Golden Do-It Book*. New York: Golden Press, 1960.

Dow, Emily. *Toys, Toddlers and Tantrums*. New York: M. Barrows, 1962.

Fielding-Jones, F. *Parent's Magazine Family Fun Book*. New York: Parent's Magazine Press, 1965. Paperback: Pocket Books, 1968.

Fletcher, H. J. *The Big Book of Things to Do and Make*. New York: Random House, 1961.

Franklin, A. *Home Play and Play Equipment*. Children's Bureau Publication #238, U.S. Department of Health, Education and Welfare. Reprinted 1966. Paperback.

Handbook of Recreation. Children's Bureau Publication #231, U.S. Department of Health, Education and Welfare, 1960. Revised 1969. Paperback.

Hartley, R., and Goldenson, R. *The Complete Book of Children's Play*. New York: Thomas Y. Crowell, 1963.

Johnson, June. *838 Ways to Amuse a Child: Crafts, Hobbies and Creative Ideas for the Child from Six to Twelve*. New York: Collier Books, 1962. Paperback.

Matterson, Elizabeth M. *Play and Playthings for the Preschool Child*. Baltimore: Penguin Books, 1965. Paperback.

Newgold, B. *Newgold's Guide to Modern Hobbies, Arts, and Crafts*. New York: David McKay, 1960.

Parker, C. *Your Child Can Be Happy in Bed: Over 200 Ways Children Can Entertain Themselves*. New York: Thomas Y. Crowell, 1962.

Peter, J., ed. *McCall's Giant Golden Make-It Book*. New York: Golden Press, 1961.

Quinn, V. *50 Card Games for Children*. Racine, Wis.: Whitman Publishing Co., 1966. Paperback.

Saunders, Everett. Whitman Creative Art Books. Racine, Wis.: Whitman Publishing Co., 1966–67. (Titles in series include *Painting, First Book; Painting, Second Book; Painting, Third Book; Paper Art; Print Art;* and *Stitchery*.)

Schwartz, Alvin. *How to Fly a Kite, Catch a Fish, Grow a Flower and Other Activities for You and Your Child*. New York: Macmillan, 1965. Paperback ed. New York: Pocket Books, 1968.

The Rainy Day Book for Housebound Families. New York: Trident Press, 1968. Paperback ed. New York: Pocket Books, 1969.

Withers, C. *A Treasury of Games.* New York: Grosset & Dunlap, 1964.

Suggested Play Materials

This section lists some materials and playthings which are appropriate for periods of free play and free time overseen by child care workers. It is meant simply to be suggestive, not comprehensive. Nor should a worker expect to have all these materials on hand—it is a rare budget which could accommodate such a long list. Also, which ones are appropriate for any group or individual depends upon a number of factors which the worker must take into consideration when he decides what to make available. (These materials are focused somewhat on younger, preadolescent children.) The materials in the list are categorized according to the general function served, although a material may also be relevant to other areas as well. Games and crafts listed in the first section of this appendix are not relisted here.

Materials by Category

Dramatic and fantasy play
  Blocks (wooden, hollow, cardboard, Styrofoam)
  Dollhouse
  Dolls (with clothes and equipment)
  Equipment for housekeeping play (toy stove, ironing board, etc.)
  Old clothes, wigs, and jewelry for dress-up
  Puppets
  Toy animals (rubber, wooden, stuffed)
  Toy cars, trucks, trains, planes, etc.
  Toy telephone, cash register

Educational and construction toys
  Alphabet and number boards (magnetic, flannel)
  Beads
  Books
  Construction toys (Lego, Tog'l, Tinker Toys, Lincoln Logs, Flexagons, etc.)
  Jigsaw puzzles
  Lacing boards and cards

Magnets
Nesting boxes, kegs, etc.
Parquetry and mosaic block sets
Put-together toys (plastic gears, nuts and bolts, interlocking blocks, etc.)
Stacking toys
Expressive and sensory play
Chalk
Charcoal
Clay (real clay, commercial Play Dough, homemade play dough)
Collage materials (scraps)
Crayons
Felt-nib markers
Paints (watercolors, temperas, finger paint, etc.)
Rhythm-band instruments
Sandbox
Soap (soap-painting, bubble-blowing)
Water-play table

Play equipment for physical exercise
Balance beam
Ball
Baton
Bowling (indoor set)
Chinning bar
Frisbee
Hula hoop
Indoor gym (for climbing and sliding)
Inner tube
Pogo stick
Punching toys
Ringtoss
Rocking boat
Rocking horse
Roller skates
Scooter
Stilts
Tricycle
Tumbling mat
Wagon
Wheelbarrow

Home Scrap Materials

Aluminum plates
Bags
Bottle caps
Bottles (wine, soda, detergent, etc.)
Boxes (salt cartons, matchboxes, shoe boxes, cylindrical boxes, plastic boxes, cigar boxes, etc.)

Buttons
Cans (coffee, frozen juice, etc.)
Clothespins
Corks
Doilies
Dowels
Egg cartons and liners
Egg shells

Feathers
Foil
Greeting cards
Hangers
Inner tubes
Jar rings
Jewelry (old)
Leaves
Linoleum
Magazines
Material scraps (felt, sheets, leather, burlap, etc.)
Milk cartons
Newspapers
Nipples
Packing materials
Paper cups
Paper plates
Paper towels and rolls
Pipe cleaners
Ribbons
Rickrack
Sawdust

Screening
Seeds
Sequins
Shells
Shirt cardboards
Soap
Socks
Sponges
Spools
Stamps (cancelled)
Stockings
Stones
Straws
String
Tableware (plastic)
Thread
Thumbtacks
Tissue paper
Toothpicks
Wallpaper
Walnut shells
Wire
Yarn

Miscellaneous Supplies

The following, in conjunction with saved home scrap materials, can assure appropriate supplies for many craft projects.

Blunt scissors
Cellophane tape
Compass
Construction paper
Crayons
Decorations (glitter, gummed stars)
Glue

Masking tape
Mucilage
Newsprint
Oak tag
Paints (watercolor, tempera, poster)
Paper clips
Pencils

Plaster of Paris	Stapler
Punch	String
Reinforcements	Tracing paper
Rubber bands	Wheat paste (for paper-
Rubber cement	mache)
Ruler	

Sources of Play Supplies and Equipment

Catalogues. Many commercial plaything manufacturers publish catalogues which can be obtained by writing to the company. Even if workers cannot place direct orders themselves, these catalogues can supply ideas for play and use of materials. Some of the better-known of these are:

American Handicrafts Company (stores located in many cities)
Childcraft Education Corporation, Post Office Box 94, Bayonne, New Jersey
Childcraft Equipment Company, 155 East Twenty-third Street, New York, New York 10010
Childplay, 43 East Nineteenth Street, New York, New York
Community Playthings, Rifton, New York 12471
Creative Playthings, Princeton, New Jersey 08540
Fisher-Price Toys, East Aurora, New York 14052
Sifo Toys, Department S-24-8M, Minneapolis, Minnesota 55411

Volunteers. Child care workers might express the opinion to volunteers that they think the children might benefit more in the long run from donations of play and game equipment than from the surfeit of parties at holiday time.

Community sources. A bit of judicious inquiry in the community might reveal to the worker sources of scrap or leftover material that would be beneficial for the unit activity program; for example, interior decorating stores will often save wallpaper sample books; lumber yards, scraps of wood, etc. Before soliciting however, it would be wise for the worker to clear with supervisors regarding agency policy for this.

Scraps from the home. Fruitful sources of materials for activities can come not only from within the institution or agency but also from home, where watching and saving yield many scrap materials that can be readily adapted into activity fun.

Suggested Reading

by George M. Cohen

Index

Suggested Reading

Child Development and Theory

Here is a list of several leading contributions to the basic understanding of the dynamics and landmarks in child development. They are useful to the worker as a foundation in developing his approaches to children.

Erikson, Erik H. *Childhood and Society*. New York: W. W. Norton, 1963.
Fraiberg, Selma. *The Magic Years*. New York: Charles Scribner's Sons, 1959.
Freud, Anna. *The Ego and the Mechanisms of Defense*. New York: International Universities Press, 1946.
_____. *Normality and Pathology in Children*. New York: International Universities Press, 1955.
Haimowitz, M. L., and Haimowitz, N., eds. *Human Development: Selected Readings*. New York: Thomas Y. Crowell, 1966.
Maier, Henry. *Three Theories of Child Development*. New York and London: Harper & Row, 1969.
Murphy, Lois. *The Widening World of Childhood: Paths Toward Mastery*. New York: Basic Books, 1962.
Piaget, Jean. *Play, Dreams and Imitation in Childhood*. New York: Norton, 1952.
Stone, L. Joseph, and Church, Joseph. *Childhood and Adolescence*. New York: Random House, 1957.

Background and Case Studies

Here are some descriptions of, or observations in, treatment settings. Some of them include studies of actual children who have been cared for in such settings. From the latter the worker can get a flavor of the long view of the history of a child as opposed to the day-to-day management with which he himself must necessarily be concerned.

Bettelheim, Bruno. *Love Is Not Enough*. Glencoe, Ill.: Free Press, 1950.
————. *Truants from Life: The Rehabilitation of Emotionally Disturbed Children*. Glencoe, Ill.: Free Press, 1955.
————. *The Empty Fortress*. New York: Free Press, 1967.
Mayer, Morris Fritz. "The Parental Figures in Residential Treatment." *Social Service Review* 34 (1960): 273–85.
Polsky, Howard W. *Cottage Six: The Social System of Delinquent Boys in Residential Treatment*. New York: John Wiley and Sons, 1962.
Redl, Fritz, and Wineman, David. *The Aggressive Child*. Glencoe, Ill.: Free Press, 1957, pp. 17–250.
Rubin, Theodore. *Lisa and David*. New York: Macmillan, 1961.

Practice and Technique

This is not an exhaustive collection, but it is a useful representation of attitudes toward the practice of child care work and of recommendations for a variety of techniques and approaches. These books and articles are listed alphabetically, not necessarily in the order in which the worker will wish to read them.

Allen, Layman. "Rules and Freedom: Games as a Mechanism for Ego Development in Children and Adolescents." Report of Workshop F, 44th annual meeting of the American Orthopsychiatric Association, New York, 1967. Mimeographed. Obtainable from the author, 1407 Brooklyn Street, Ann Arbor, Michigan.
Babcock, Charlotte. "Having Chosen to Work with Children." Paper read for the Extension Division of the Child Therapy Program, the Institute for Psychoanalysis, Chicago, Ill., February 10, 1964. Obtainable from Dr. Babcock at the Western Psychiatric Institute and Clinic, 3811 O'Hara Street, Pittsburgh, Pa. 15213.
Bettelheim, Bruno, and Sylvester, Emmy. "A Therapeutic Milieu." *American Journal of Orthopsychiatry* 18: 191–206.
Broten, Alton M. *Houseparents in Children's Institutions: A Discussion Guide*. Chapel Hill: University of North Carolina Press, 1962.
Burmeister, Eva. *The Professional Houseparent*. New York: Columbia University Press, 1960.
————. *Tough Times and Tender Moments in Child Care Work*. New York and London: Columbia University Press, 1967.

Carbonara, Nancy Trevorrow. *Techniques for Observing Normal Child Behavior*. Pittsburgh: University of Pittsburgh Press, 1961.

Cumming, John, and Cumming, Elaine. *Ego and Milieu: Theory and Practice of Environmental Therapy*. New York: Atherton Press, 1962.

Ferster, C. B., and Simons, Jeanne. "Behavior Therapy with Children." *Psychological Record* 16: 65–71.

Flint, Betty Margaret. *The Child and the Institution: A Study of Deprivation and Recovery*. Toronto: University of Toronto Press, 1966.

Ginott, Haim G. *Between Parent and Child*. New York: Macmillan, 1965.

Grossbard, Hyman. *Cottage Parents: What They Have to Be, Know, and Do*. New York: Child Welfare League of America, 1960.

Konopka, Gisela. *Group Work in the Institution: A Modern Challenge*. New York: Association Press, 1970.

Long, Nicholas J.; Morse, William C.; and Newman, Ruth G., eds. *Conflict in the Classroom: The Education of Emotionally Disturbed Children*. Belmont, Calif.: Wadsworth, 1965.

Mayer, Morris Fritz. *A Guide for Child Care Workers*. New York: Child Welfare League of America, 1958.

Mowrer, O. Hobart. "The Behavior Therapies with Special Reference to Modeling and Imitation." *American Journal of Psychotherapy* 20: 439–61.

Paradise, Robert J. "The Factor of Timing in the Addition of New Members to Established Groups." *Child Welfare* 47: 524–29.

Redl, Fritz. "The Impact of Game Ingredients on Children's Play Behavior." In *Fourth Josiah Macy Foundation Conference on Group Processes*, ed. Bertram Schaffner. New York: Josiah Macy Foundation, 1959.

Redl, Fritz, and Wineman, David. *The Aggressive Child*. Glencoe, Ill.: Free Press, 1957.

Switzer, Robert E. "Security Is a Child Care Worker." Paper given to the graduating class of the Certificate Program, Western Psychiatric Institute and Clinic, Pittsburgh, Pa., June 7, 1967. Obtainable from Dr. Switzer, Director of the Children's Division of the Menninger Foundation, Topeka, Kans.

Trieschman, Albert E.; Paradise, R. J.; and Segal, R. L. "Bedtime Management in a Children's Home." *Mental Hygiene* 51:209–20.

Trieschman, Albert E.; Whittaker, James K.; and Brendtro, Larry K. *The Other Twenty-three Hours*. Chicago: Aldine, 1969.

Vintner, Robert D., ed. *Group Work Practice*. Ann Arbor, Mich.: Campus Publishers, 1969.

Index

Acting out. *See* Behavior problems

Activities: in-between, 80; importance of, 108; lack of, for withdrawn children, 109; administration of, 203–42; unstructured, 217; overinterest in, 226

Activity materials: care of, 75–76, 170–71; care of dangerous, 172; recommended, 253–55

Activity workers: in institution, 105; in living unit, 105, 128

Administration: of institution, 195

Administrator, institutional: and change from custodial to therapeutic care, 19

Adults: outnumbering children, 88

Age: of child care workers, 3, 10; of children in institutional groups, 104; and appropriateness for activities, 224

Aggression: worker's handling of, 43–44; and prevention of injury, 63; rechannelling of, in activities, 234

Anger: in disturbed child, 42–43; first expressions of, 43; realization of, 43; on part of worker, 93, 94; between staff members, 195

Anxiety: study of effects of, xvi; child's nonrecognition of, 37; in withdrawn children, 37; masked by behavior, 38; at absence of child from group, 39; at separation

from parents, 39; reassurance by worker in case of, 39–40; caused by change, 41; process of mastery of, 41; in new kinds of play, 47; about bathing or toileting, 64; at night, 72–73; at separation from worker, 74; when worker goes off duty, 74; expressed by masturbation, 159

Approval of worker: as incentive to work on problems, 59

Assistance, activity, 240

Autonomy need: satisfaction of, 50; meeting, in daily care, 64

Background information, children's: availability to workers of, 181

Basic trust. *See* Trust

Bathing: anxiety over, 64; rituals about, 65; compromise on, 67; and withdrawn child, 67

Bedtime: anxiety over, 72; and behavior problems, 72; rituals, 72; and toys in bed, 72–73

Behavior problems: of children in treatment groups, 15, 101; expectations and limit-setting with, 53–61; institutional discipline for, 124–42 passim; medication for, 144

Boredom: as result of lack of program, 109; masturbation as result of, 159

265